MIDLIFE HEALTH

EVERY WOMAN'S GUIDE
TO FEELING GOOD

Ada P. Kahn
Linda Hughey Holt, M.D.

Facts On File Publications
New York, New York ● Oxford, England

Medical information contained in this book is general information only, and readers are advised to consult with their personal physicians about their own medical problems.

Library of Congress Cataloging-in-Publication Data

Kahn, Ada P.
  Midlife health.

  Bibliography:p.
  Includes index.
    1. Middle aged women—Health and hygiene. 2. Middle aged women—Health and Hygiene—United States—Public opinion. 3. Health surveys—United States. I. Holt, Linda Hughey. II. Title. (DNLM: 1. Health. 2. Middle age—popular works. 3. Women—popular works. WT 120 K12m)
RA778.K125 1986   613'.04244   86-19954
ISBN 0-8160-1345-4

Printed in the United States of America

10 9 8 7 6 5 4 3 2

CONTENTS

ACKNOWLEDGMENTS

Many individuals, organizations, and institutions assisted with the compilation of information in MIDLIFE HEALTH. We are particularly grateful to the alumni office, Northwestern University (Evanston) and women of the classes of 1955 and 1956; women of the Roosevelt High School (Chicago) class of June 1952; members of Women in Communications, Inc. (who were initiated into Theta Sigma Phi during the late 1940s and 1950s); physician members of the American College of Obstetricians and Gynecologists; and all others (anonymous) who participated in the Holt-Kahn survey described in the book.

We thank the following for sharing opinions and comments: Richard Allen, marketing director, Empire Blue Cross Blue Shield HMO, NY; Arthur K. Balin, M.D., Ph.D., assistant professor and associate physician at The Rockefeller University Hospital; John E. Garnett, M.D., Northwestern Memorial Hospital, Chicago; Uriel Barzel, M.D., professor of medicine, Albert Einstein College of Medicine, Bronx, NY; Timothy Bell and Rebecca Gradowski of Timothy Bell & Company, Reston, VA; Harriet Benson, Ph.D., Palo Alto, CA; Donald Bliwise, Ph.D., Sleep Disorders Center, Stanford University Medical School, Palo Alto, CA; Dr. Rosalind Cartwright, director, Sleep Disorder Center, Rush-Presbyterian-St. Luke's Medical Center, Chicago; Thora DeLey, Feminist Women's Health Center, Chico, CA; Dudley S. Dinner, M.D., director, Sleep Disorders Center, The Cleveland Clinic Foundation, Cleveland; Carol Downer, vice president, Federation of Feminist Women's Health Centers, Los Angeles; Julie Duffy, Ac.T., president, Illinois State Acupuncturists Association and Dean of Students, Midwest Center for the Study of Oriental Medicine, Chicago.

Also, Robert Dunbar, M.S.J., Damariscotta, ME; William Dunbar, D.N., C.A., director, Midwest Center for the Study of Oriental Medicine, Chicago;

Carol E. Goodman, M.D., Department of Physical Medicine and Rehabilitation, Ochsner Clinic and Medical Foundation, New Orleans, LA; Sadja Greenwood, M.D., San Francisco; Dido Hasper, executive director, Feminist Women's Health Center, Chico, CA; Robert Heaney, M.D., Creighton University School of Medicine, Omaha, NE; Hal Higdon, Michigan City, IN; Charlene Karns, Chicago; Taube Kaufman, M.S.W., C.W.S., founder and president, Combined Families Association of America, Inc., Northbrook, IL; Charles R. Kleeman, M.D., director emeritus, Center for Health Enhancement, University of California, Los Angeles Medical Center; Angelo A. Licata, M.D., Ph.D., Department of Endocrinology, The Cleveland Clinic Foundation; Ann Marcou, Y-Me Breast Cancer Support Program, Homewood, IL; Robert Marcus, M.D., director, Aging Study Unit, VA Medical Center, Palo Alto, CA, and associate professor of medicine, Stanford University; Richard B. Mazess, Ph.D., Department of Medical Physics, University of Wisconsin, Madison, WI.

Also, Mary McMahon, A.C.S., Department of Psychiatry, Evanston Hospital, Evanston, IL; Marion Mosely, The Cleveland Clinic Foundation, Cleveland; Gregory R. Mundy, M.D., head, Division of Endocrinology and Metabolism, Department of Medicine, University of Texas Health Science Center, San Antonio; Donald A. Nagel, M.D., professor and head, Division of Orthopedic Surgery, Stanford University School of Medicine; Yvonne Parnes, R.N., nurse practitioner, Community Health Program of Queens, NY; Phyllis Perlman, R.N., M.S., Bayshore, NY; Marvin Posner, M.D., medical director, Community Health Plan of Suffolk, Hauppauge, NY, and associate professor, Department of Community and Preventive Medicine, State University of New York at Stony Brook; Robert R. Recker, M.D., Creighton University School of Medicine, Omaha, NE.

Also, Domeena Renshaw, M.D., professor, Department of Psychiatry, and director, Loyola Sexual Dysfunction Training Clinic, Loyola University of Chicago; Anne Rudolph, Chicago; Will G. Ryan, M.D., director, Osteoporosis Center, Rush-Presbyterian-St. Luke's Medical Center, Chicago; Everett L. Smith, Ph.D., director, Biogerontology Laboratory, Department of Preventive Medicine, University of Wisconsin, Madison; Jeanne Wielage Smith, Ph.D., coordinator of the Academic Reentry Program and instructor, applied behavioral sciences, University of California at Davis; Robert M. Swartz, M.D., F.A.C.S., Arlington Heights, IL; Linda V. VanHorn, Ph.D., R.D., spokesperson for the American Dietetic Association and associate professor, Department of Community Health and Preventive Medicine, Northwestern University School of Medicine, Chicago; Gabrielle Woloshin, M.D., Highland Park, IL; Rachel Yeager, Ph.D., Human Performance Laboratory, West Virginia University, Morgantown, WV; and Patricia Zak, Chicago.

We thank the following organizations and institutions for their contributions of information: Aging Study Unit, VA Medical Center, Palo Alto, CA;

American Cancer Society, NY; American College of Obstetricians and Gynecologists, Washington, D.C.; American Podiatric Medical Association, Washington, D.C.; The Arthritis Foundation, Atlanta, GA; Federation of Feminist Women's Health Centers; Illinois Governor's Council on Physical Fitness, Springfield, IL; Midwest Center for the Study of Oriental Medicine, Chicago; National Dairy Council; Osteoporosis Center, Rush-Presbyterian-St. Luke's Medical Center, Chicago; Saint Francis Hospital, Evanston, IL; and the Southern Medical Association.

Analysis for the Holt-Kahn survey was performed by Harry Nelson, Vogelback Computing Center, Northwestern University, Evanston, IL.

INTRODUCTION

"Do you still get your periods?" "Do you worry about getting pregnant at our age?" "Do you get hot flashes?" "Do you take estrogens?" "Do you worry about getting osteoporosis?" "Do you take calcium supplements?"

These are questions that women our age ask. As a 51-year-old medical writer and health educator (Ada P. Kahn) and a gynecologist (Linda Hughey Holt), we are expected to come up with good answers about the best ways to progress through what for years has been referred to as "the change of life." Trying to answer such questions in an informative and positive way led to our writing this book. We found that there *isn't* a lot to read about women's midlife health. Because menopause is not a life-threatening condition, it hasn't received extensive coverage in medical and popular publications. And we were surprised to find only one chapter about menopause in many gynecology textbooks, and that one is generally placed just before the chapter on senility! This concerns us, because women now spend approximately one-third of their lives in the postmenopausal state.

To find out what today's women are thinking and doing about midlife health, we mailed questionnaires to 2,000 women between the ages of 45 and 60. Of the 967 respondents (nearly 50%!), some were high school and college classmates and non-physician colleagues in a professional society. Fifty-two were gynecologists in the same age group. Of all respondents, nearly half (41.3%) were either 50 or 51 years old, which is the average age for menopause in the United States today.

Of the 967 respondents, 72.8% were married, 4.7% were widowed, 9.7% were single, and 12.9% were divorced; 26.3% were grandmothers. Of the respondents, 69.3% no longer menstruate. The highest percentage (15.4%) reported having their last period at age 50 (the range was 48-51).

The women's answers are summarized throughout this book. They also gave us comments on many topics relating to midlife health that we want you to "overhear." Thus we regard this book as a conversation among women. Perhaps you have problems that you haven't even discussed with your friends. Are you different from most women your age? You'll find out here.

This book also will give you some basis with which to compare your own symptoms* and attitudes, and may help you determine if your symptoms are usual or unusual, and whether they warrant medical attention. You *can* deal successfully with many symptoms yourself.

Women in our survey group have had their share of medical problems, too. Thirteen percent have high blood pressure, 2.2% have heart disease, and 1.3% have diabetes. 29.7% have had hysterectomies, 13.4% do not have their ovaries, and 18% had breast surgery. Of the group, 18% smoke. (We hope you stop soon.)

Despite a few bad cards dealt by life, today's 50-year-old is doing better than ever. She's busy, active, involved, and sees at least a third of her life still ahead of her. 71.3% of our respondents work full time (80.8% reported working full time or part time).

To a nifty-50, menopause is a natural step along the road of life. Menopause happens at an age when we're old enough to know what's going on and still young enough to do something about it.

As you approach, enter, or complete your "change of life" and grow older, do you know what to expect? You can talk with friends and relatives and gather some information—as well as myths. You can talk with your doctor and learn more. But you may also be told "Don't worry about it," or "Most women your age can expect these problems." Can you? Should you?

You picked up this book because you have greater expectations for your future health than your mothers and grandmothers may have had. You want to know more about the best ways to take care of yourself and your health as you grow older. You want more information about the basic health issues you will face as you grow past your childbearing years.

This is an easy-to-understand guidebook for midlife and beyond. It will give you a practical combination of medical and self-help information that you may be able to use right away and in years ahead. It will help you to use our medical-care system wisely and most economically. It will give you ideas from other women your age, including women gynecologists, who face similar issues. Finally, it will help you prepare yourself for midlife and beyond in healthier ways.

---

*By using the word *symptom* throughout the book, we don't mean to imply that menopause is a "disease" through which women must "suffer." In fact, as you'll see, we believe that menopause (and beyond) should be a positive, enjoyable time for women. We use the word *symptom* more generally as just an indication of an underlying physical condition.

In many ways, women of the same age are very much alike, whether we have careers in the business world, or are volunteers in community activities, or focus most of our attention on the home. In our forties, fifties, and beyond, we all face the same issues—our own menopause, our husband's midlife problems, perhaps loss of our husband to death or divorce, and coping with single life, our children's teen years, children leaving home, our own career choices, and aging parents.

Our attitudes about how our body works are probably similar. Many of us learned about menstruation from the little pink booklets produced by a manufacturer of popular feminine napkins. Perhaps the title was "The Stork Didn't Bring You."

Many of us say that sexual activity was "saved" for the man we loved until after marriage (or we didn't talk about it). As brides, we delved into the then-popular manuals about ideal marriages to learn more than we had learned from school health classes. We may have enrolled in a childbirth education class before the first baby arrived. Perhaps our husbands were among the first group of fathers to participate in training for childbirth.

Some of us grew up thinking that a woman's life cycle began with menstrual periods and ended when the childbearing years were over: the Big 50! But it's not all over! Give yourself a new "warranty" by taking good care of yourself in a society in which one of the greatest compliments you can hear is "You don't look your age!"

Booklets, manuals, and support groups helped you through earlier important phases of your life. Now, there seem to be few guidebooks and sources of information to use during your climacteric, the phases of life that include the years just before menstruation ceases, the time when menstruation ceases, and the years afterward. This book may be just what you have been seeking.

1
WHAT MENOPAUSE MEANS

"Put warnings in your book against easy acceptance of gynecologists' prescriptions for drugs as though menopause is a disease."

"I never had any problems. Must admit, it's nice, now, not to have to worry about packing a supply of Kotex when I go on vacation."

"I hope someone sometime would capture doctors' attention to make them realize there is more to menopause than cessation of periods and hot flashes. The body is experiencing hormonal changes that can't help but have more far-reaching results than the two criteria my doctor says are all there is to menopause."

"I'd like to see a serious description of variations in menopause; how long it lasts for most women; physical and mental changes. Describe real problems some women have as well as the easy time we're all supposed to have."

"What should the average, healthy woman expect? All I seem to hear about are the people who don't experience any symptoms or the ones who have a really bad time—no in-between."

You may have heard the phrase "change of life" first from your grandmother, mother, or aunt. If you asked what the "change" meant, the responses may have influenced your thinking about menopause as well as yourself as an older woman. Did their ideas stay with you? Do you agree now with their opinions?

Probably your expectations are higher than theirs. There are good reasons for more positive thinking. We live in a high-technology world. They struggled to exist. Although we also face the inevitable, we have better tools to cope with the cards life deals to us.

1

Still, many women are somewhat uneasy about menopause. Despite the fact that the Jane Fondas and Joan Collinses of the world assure us that we, too, can look ravishing at 45 or 50 (with the help of careful diet, hours of exercise, makeup artists, and plastic surgeons), most of us are well aware that for every ravishing 50-year-old (who started out as a ravishing 20-year-old), there are thousands of women concerned about facial wrinkles and bulging hips.

> *"My only real complaint is the weight gain and more matronly mid-section I seem to have acquired. I feel it's due to the estrogen."*

During the forties and fifties, certain universal physical events occur in women:

- Estrogen production declines.
- Ovulation stops.
- Pituitary hormones FSH (follicle stimulating hormone) and LH (luteinizing hormone) rise dramatically.

Physical changes that women commonly notice include:

- Hot flashes.
- Dry skin.
- Vaginal dryness.
- Weight gain, particularly around the mid-section.
- Mood swings (crying spells, outbursts of anger, depression).
- Increase in skin tags and darkening of moles, "blotches" on skin.
- Bladder symptoms (loss of urine with coughing, sneezing).
- Changes in sex drive (either increase or decrease).

In addition to changes women notice, a change they do not notice is an acceleration of bone loss that can lead to fractures later in life.

Sound depressing? Not all of these changes are inevitable, and in fact, it is unclear whether some of them relate to hormonal changes or whether they are simply the result of the aging process. Each of these changes will be discussed in detail in the chapters to follow. We hope our discussion wll help you to change what can be changed and adjust gracefully to what cannot be changed.

COMING TO TERMS

Just what does "change of life" mean? What did it mean to previous generations? What does it or will it mean for you?

Doctors use a variety of words to describe this time of life.

If you are still in your forties, your doctor may use the terms "premenopausal," "perimenopausal," or "beginning your climacteric" when discussing your health.

If you are in your fifties and over, your doctor may use the term "menopausal" or "postmenopausal."

How do these terms describe an eventful segment of your life?

Climacteric

Climacteric and *menopause* are not synonymous, because climacteric refers to a time span and menopause refers to a specific event.

How do you know that you are on the climacteric track? You may not even know it until something dramatic happens—or doesn't happen—such as a missed period. In earlier years you might have worried about being pregnant—and that's still a possibility—but now the missed period probably means that you are entering a new phase of your life.

The climacteric (some writers use the word *climacterium*) is the medical term for an approximately 10– to 15–year span of life. These are the years from about ages 35–40 to 50–55 when a woman goes from the reproductive to the nonreproductive stage.

During the climacteric, your body's hormonal production decreases, your ovaries gradually stop producing and releasing eggs, and your menstrual cycles change and monthly flow ceases. After age 35 to 40, your hormonal levels gradually decline, and in the late forties, levels decline sharply. For some women, the climacteric span is shorter than 10 years. For others it is longer. Ten years seems about average.

There is no specific time for the climacteric to occur. For some it is completed during the forties. On the other hand, many women continue to have regular menstrual periods into and throughout their fifties.

Physicians generally divide the climacteric into several clinical phases: premenopause, perimenopause, menopause, and postmenopause. By understanding the features of each phase, you may be able to anticipate what will occur and when you may expect certain changes.

Premenopause

For many women, the stage known as premenopause usually begins some time after age 40. At this time, some women notice that their periods are irregular. Other women's periods, however, are still regular. Both situations are normal.

Your doctor may tell you that you are no longer ovulating, and if your menstrual cycle is irregular, you may be premenopausal. You may go through a span of months or even years of transition. There are no clear-cut guidelines about how long the transition lasts.

Perimenopause

The time closest to the last menstrual period is the perimenopause. Many women go for several months at a time without having a period. Some women think they have had their last period because they haven't had one in many months, or even a year, and then, surprise! There it is again.

Menopause

The date of your final menstrual period is your formal date of menopause, just in case you want an anniversary to remember. However, you won't know that it was your last period until you haven't had another one.

Just as you did in earlier years, continue to write down the dates of your periods so that you remember when your last one occurred. Then you'll know your menopause date, just as you remembered the date of your first period, a long time ago.

Interestingly, although the age at which young women begin to menstruate has become earlier throughout the generations, it seems that the age of menopause has changed only slightly over hundreds of years. One researcher analyzed historical data and suggested that in ancient times, menopause occurred at age 40; in the years 1500 to 1830, age 45; and in 1948, 48. (Leon Speroff, Robert H. Glass, Nathan G. Kase, *Clinical Gynecologic Endocrinology and Infertility*, 3rd ed. [Baltimore: Williams and Wilkins, 1983].)

In the United States, the usual age of menopause is between 48 and 55 years, with the median age of 51.4. The average age in our survey group was 50. (The range was 48 to 51.)

When will your menopause occur?

Can you predict when your own menopause will occur? Probably not. Many physicians say that there is no relationship between the age of the menarche (beginning of menstrual periods) and your age at menopause. Some people once thought that an early start meant an early finish, or a late start meant a late finish. In studies early in this century, researchers relied on women's recollections of how old they were when their periods started. Some recollections were only within a five-year range, and this made the overall correlation somewhat unreliable. Now, researchers are not sure about the early/late start and the early/late finish.

WHAT INFLUENCES AGE OF MENOPAUSE? There are a number of areas that are unclear because no researchers have yet collected data on them. These include effects, if any, of marital status, oral contraceptive use, and childbearing on the age of menopause. It is difficult to correlate these factors with menopause because various factors interrelate to bring about menopause. However, some research indicates an *association* between some of these factors, but not *causation*.

Once researchers thought that a rapid succession of pregnancies and childbirths and continuous lactation exhausted a woman's reproductive capabilities and brought on early menopause. Other researchers later refuted this idea. Some said that more pregnancies caused a later menopause. Others said that there is no relationship between number of pregnancies and age at menopause.

Also, some researchers once thought that a woman's age at her last pregnancy had an effect on when menopause would occur. Now, it seems that there is no relationship between your age during your last pregnancy (or number of pregnancies) and the age at which your menopause occurs. Of course, women who go through premature menopause can't have children in their forties, and women who have children in their forties are going to have late menopause! Other researchers have compared groups of un-married women with married women, and women who had children compared with women who never had children. There were no significant differences in age at menopause between these various groups.

It does appear that slender women generally experience menopause earlier than obese women, and that athletic women experience it before more sedentary women.

Researchers have even considered whether climate and altitude in-fluence age of menopause. One group speculated that women living in tropi-cal climates have their menopause at 30 to 40 years, while in temperate climates it is at age 45 to 60. Later, another group refuted this claim and said that while nutrition and general health factors may influence menopause, climate per se seems to have little effect.

Socioeconomic influences One factor that may affect age of menopause is socioeconomic conditions that may affect one's level of nutri-tion, education, and overall health. Women whose mothers and sisters have a particularly early or late menopause may show a similar tendency. Dietary factors such as a high-meat, high-fat diet may prolong periods. Hormone use can artificially produce regular bleeding, although such bleeding episodes are not true "periods."

Effects of oral contraceptives Some researchers believe that use of oral contraceptives may affect the age of menopause, but most studies show no correlation between menopause and Pill use.

How does the doctor know when you are menopausal?

Around age 40 to 50, your doctor will ask you questions about the regularity of your periods, and if you have any of the symptoms often associated with decreased ovarian function. Based on your answers, your doctor will be able to determine if you are near your menopause.

Additionally, to help reinforce the diagnosis, your doctor may use vaginal cytology (a microscopic study of the cells from your vagina) to estimate your estrogen levels. However, interpretations of estrogen production from Pap smears are not conclusive because factors such as vaginal infections, tissue sensitivity, and the effects of certain medications and disease may influence the findings.

To evaluate your hormonal status, a doctor may take blood samples to look at levels of two pituitary hormones called LH (luteinizing hormone) and FSH (follicle-stimulating hormone). Levels of these hormones are elevated after menopause, but tend to be low in women whose periods have temporarily stopped due to stress or weight loss. Obviously, pregnancy must be considered as a possible reason why the periods have stopped. It is important to make a pregnancy diagnosis early enough to offer a midlife woman such options as genetic testing. In many cases, no special testing is necessary if body symptoms are typical of menopause and pregnancy is unlikely.

Some types of pregnancy tests can be "false positive" after menopause, so before you panic, seek consultation from a knowledgeable doctor if you do get a positive value. Also, abnormal pregnancies (early miscarriages, ectopics) can give false negative readings. If you are in pain or "feel" pregnant, seek medical advice.

Premature Menopause

If menopause occurs before age 35, physicians say it is "premature." Sometimes this is normal. Hereditary factors influence age of menopause, and in some families, women reach menopause early. However, if you are in your thirties and cease to have periods, don't just assume that it is early menopause. Amenorrhea (absence of menstruation) may be due to disorders of your hypothalamus or pituitary gland. Be sure to ask your doctor to investigate all possible causes if your periods stop at an early age.

Induced Menopause

Surgical removal of the ovaries will cause early menopause.

Approximately 29.7% of our questionnaire respondents have had hysterectomies. Many respondents referred to their surgeries:

> "I'd like to see a discussion in your book of the emotional problems resulting from a hysterectomy. I wonder if I am the only one who had problems for several years."

> "I was concerned about the aftereffects of a surgical menopause two years ago, but I've found no physical or mental differences except hot flashes the first few months and slight loss of suppleness in ligaments."

> "Even though I had my ovaries left in when I had my hysterectomy, I still experienced a change in my body. My doctor said there would be none; however, there is a change in my skin, hair, and emotions."

Excessive irradiation of the ovaries will bring about an early menopause. Early menopause sometimes results from levels of X rays used in treatment of abdominal cancers (Hodgkin's disease or kidney cancers). However, this will not happen from diagnostic X rays.

Also, chronic disease can bring about ovarian failure, but lack of menstruation together with extended illness is more likely to be a result of suppression of the hypothalamus (a gland in the brain) than to failure of the ovaries.

Delayed Menopause

Some women continue to menstruate regularly after age 55. For some this is perfectly normal, but it may indicate a symptom to ask your doctor about. There are many possibilities for extended menstruation. For example, a woman may still have periods because she is taking hormones, because she has a type of cell tumor that secretes estrogen and thus induces menstruation, or because she has a type of uterine growth that results in bleeding.

Certain diseases are associated with either early or late menopause. Diseases associated with an early menopause are "vulvar dystrophy," a group of vulvar conditions often characterized by delicate or raw, itchy vaginal tissues and osteoporosis. Diseases associated with a late menopause include diabetes, cancer of the uterus, cancer of the breast, cancer of the cervix, fibroids, and polyps. A common denominator of these conditions is obesity and high estrogen levels. You'll read more about estrogen levels and their overall effects on your body in later chapters.

Postmenopausal

You may classify yourself as postmenopausal if you haven't had a period for at least one year. The phrase "change of life" really applies throughout the female life cycle. Changes are ongoing—long before "the big change." Many women who rarely thought about physical changes since menstruation began now look at themselves and their symptoms very analytically. To give you a better perspective from which to look at your own health around menopause, the next two chapters explain common symptoms and why they result from certain physical changes that occur at this time. There *is* something that you can do about many of the symptoms. You'll find helpful hints to make yourself more informed and more comfortable. Many of these hints for feeling and looking better have been gathered from comments in our survey.

"Menopause was not the dreaded experience I had always heard about. My periods became farther apart and finally stopped. Didn't have hot flashes or abnormal depression. Frankly, it is lovely not to have the monthly mess."

"I think working women have less trauma because they have less time to focus on themselves. They are too busy to worry about it."

"Keeping a cool head is the main thing. It's all much easier than I expected."

"Women should not fear menopause and they won't if they are educated on the subject. Women my age grew up on old wives' tales."

"Be aware of it, but try to forget about it. Keep very active physically and mentally so you feel good. Menopause is a completely natural event in the life of a woman. Frankly, I welcome it. I feel stronger and more vigorous than ever before and there's much less worry about pregnancy, etc. I even look better . . . so there!"

2

"NORMAL" SYMPTOMS AND HOW TO FEEL BETTER

"I only had a few hot flashes over a period of six months, and then my periods stopped. No other symptoms. When I think about some of the stories I hear from other women at the health club, I wonder if I've missed out on some of the menopausal experience!"

"It's a misery, yet kind of funny (if you can laugh through your sweat and tears)!"

"I really feel much too much emphasis is placed on menopause. If one accepts this as a natural period of one's life and keeps occupied and vital, it's not really a problem. I find 'hot flashes' have diminished by limiting sugar intake."

"Is this normal?" is a frequent question asked in doctors' offices. Most of the time the answer is yes. Menopausal and postmenopausal women have a wide range of "normal" symptoms.

Also, many women ask, "What can I expect with menopause?" This is a difficult question to answer in a specific way because symptoms of "the change" vary from woman to woman, just as length of eyelashes varies among us.

Following is a "shopping list" of common symptoms that many women experience to different degrees. You may experience one or more of them, or perhaps none at all. Knowing about them may reassure you that what you are experiencing is indeed "normal."

- Hot flashes
- Irregular periods and premenstrual syndrome (PMS)
- Vaginal dryness
- Stress incontinence

- Weight gain
- Breast enlargement or diminution
- Skin and hair changes; increase in moles
- Varicose veins
- Vision changes
- Sleep disturbances
- Bone changes

Some women have no symptoms of menopause. Their periods just stop. Other women have irregular periods for a year or more, or may have a lighter or heavier flow until their periods stop.

According to the National Institutes of Health, about 80% of women experience mild or no menopausal symptoms; about 20% report symptoms severe enough for the women to seek medical attention.

HOT FLASHES ARE THE MOST COMMON SYMPTOM

"Turtleneck sweaters are shelved for several years!"

"I have heard that if you just work hard you won't notice you are going through this time of life. The harder I worked the more and harder my hot flashes were. How can you sleep through one? What happens is you lose lots of hours of sleep, sometimes all night."

In the Holt-Kahn survey, 63.3% complained of hot flashes: 16% ranked them as severe and 47.3% ranked theirs as "mild."

Other researchers report a higher incidence of women seeking medical assistance for menopausal symptoms, particularly for hot flashes. According to the *Journal of the American Geriatrics Society* (September 1981), 75% of all postmenopausal women experience these symptoms, with 45% seeking medical treatment for them.

Some women may experience hot flashes in their sleep, during stress, during temperature changes, or "out of the blue."

"I am astounded at the horrific life-disruption night hot flashes cause, and my OB's casual attitude. These things have been around all this time and no one has done the research needed to explain and eradicate them."

Hot flashes may be one of the first menopausal symptoms a woman notices, even before her periods stop. They may continue after she no longer menstruates. Some women have hot flashes several times a day, once a week, or less frequently.

For most women, hot flashes are self-limiting symptoms and disappear without any treatment. However, there is some disagreement between the experts and women themselves concerning when hot flashes stop. According to a report in the *Journal of the American Geriatric Society* (September 1982), they usually stop within one to five years, yet some women report that they had hot flashes over a ten-year period. Many respondents in our survey reported hot flashes long after menstruation stopped.

Hot flashes appear in many durations and intensities. Some women say they "think they have them," while others are quite sure. Many women just think that they are warmer than others around them. Those whose sleep is disturbed during the night by sudden, severe perspiration have no doubt about having hot flashes. Although hot flashes are not a threat to health, they can be a temporary threat to a woman's comfort and confidence.

Different women find different things bothersome about hot flashes. Typical complaints are:

- Suddenly perspiring, then feeling chilly, clammy, or breaking out in a cold sweat
- Waking up at night drenched in sweat (if this happens often, a woman becomes exhausted, irritable, and depressed)
- Ruining clothes from perspiration
- Feeling embarrassed at flushing and shivering with no control
- Being intolerant of heat or cold: Many women find their bodies unable to deal comfortably with even slight variations in temperature

What Happens During a Hot Flash?

"It is possible for your temperature to rise to 104 degrees Farenheit when you have a hot flash, and it is very uncomfortable and devastating, especially when you are in the public eye."

A hormone known as luteinizing hormone (LH) rises after menopause. Before menopause it is the substance that helps trigger ovulation. LH "surges" seem to set off hot flashes by dilating surface blood vessels.

Hormonal changes associated with the hot flash may also be due to nerve activity in the hypothalamic area that controls temperature and anterior pituitary function.

Most women who have experienced a hot flash say that an unpredictable, sudden feeling of warmth occurs on the face, chest, or entire body. The woman's face may become flushed, and patches of redness may appear on her chest, back, shoulders, and upper arms. As her body temperature readjusts, she may perspire profusely and have a cold, clammy sensation. Episodes may last from seconds to minutes.

As sweat evaporates, the body temperature decreases, which sometimes causes chills or a cold, clammy sensation.

Twins or Hot Flashes?

In some women, increased LH and FSH levels trigger ovulation or even double ovulation, and that is why fraternal twins are born more frequently to mature mothers than to younger mothers. In most women, however, the ovaries cannot respond and the LH triggers only hot flashes.

Many women make this transition so gradually that they never have a symptom exept a very gradual lightening of menses. Other women make the transition abruptly. Some women with a sudden cessation of ovarian cyclic function have severe hot flashes. Some women with off-again, on-again ovarian function go through years of hot flashes.

"Hot Flashes" About Hot Flashes

Here are some helpful hints about hot flashes from post-menopausal women:

- Air stuffy rooms, keep a window open if you are warm, close the window if you are cold.
- Layer your clothing. A suit with a lightweight blouse gives you more flexibility than a wool dress. If you feel too warm, remove your jacket.
- Wear a cotton (or other absorbent material) blouse under a sweater Don't wear a sweater next to your skin. (You'll be more comfortable after a hot flash if you don't have wet wool next to you!)
- Put your silk blouses away for a while. You won't want to stain them with perspiration.
- If you work at a desk, get a small, desk-top fan. If you feel warm, just turn on your personal fan.
- When you have a hot flash, don't overreact. If you keep calm, no one else will pay much attention to what is happening to you.
- You can learn relaxation techniques that will help you feel in control of the situation. Most women find lack of control over hot flashes frustrating.
- Regular exercise will tone your vascular system and may help you feel better.
- Keep your weight down. Slender women seem to have less erratic estrogen production, and hence less erratic experiences with hot flashes.

When to Seek Medical Help with Hot Flashes

- If you wake up with hot flashes so often that you frequently cannot get a good night's sleep

- If hot flashes interfere with your marriage or your work
- If hot flashes make you chronically depressed and exhausted

For a discussion of treatment for hot flashes with estrogen replacement therapy, see chapter 6. Alternatives to hormones include sedatives and "anticholinergic" agents, which some women find decrease the rapid vascular changes responsible for hot flashes. You'll also find some ideas about herbal remedies recommended by women's health centers.

Generally, hot flashes are the only known menopausal symptoms directly related to LH and FSH. Most other symptoms are due to changes in sex steroids. The following section will give you a general overview of the complicated subject of hormones and how they relate to common menopausal symptoms.

OTHER SYMPTOMS ARE CAUSED BY HORMONAL CHANGES

Cyclic Hormones

Cyclic hormones influence your body shape

Prior to menopause, your pituitary gland and ovaries secrete a cyclic flow of the hormones LH and FSH. The ovaries secrete androgen, estrogen, and progesterone. Also, the adrenal glands (small glands that sit on top of the kidneys) secrete sex steroids; adrenal steroids become an increasingly important source of sex hormones in later years. Then, too, the skin and fatty tissue can convert sex hormones from androgenic (male characteristic-producing) to estrogenic (female characteristic-producing).

Sound confusing? It need not be. Keeping in mind that all of the sex steroids are closely related will help you understand the changes that occur at menopause. Think of hormones as internal "messengers" that cause body changes. The most active messengers are estrogen, progesterone, and androgen.

ESTROGEN is the name of a category of hormones that have common effects. The ovaries produce estrogens, and they are also made in the skin, adrenal glands, and fatty tissues. Estrogens are also made synthetically. Estrogen stimulates the lining of the uterus to prepare for ovulation, influences the depth and thickness of the vaginal walls, and stimulates development of the breasts. In subtle ways estrogens also affect your skin, hair, blood, liver, and bones.

PROGESTERONE is a female hormone produced by the ovaries (during pregnancy, produced by the placenta). Progesterone is the most common form of a class of hormones called progestins. Progestins change the lining of the uterus and prepare the body in many ways for pregnancy. Decreasing progesterone production prior to and during menopause may lead to symptoms of "estrogen excess," such as heavy and erratic menses.

ANDROGENS are male hormones. They can be secreted in the ovaries or the adrenal glands. Women naturally have some androgens, but if these hormones are excessive, certain "male" characteristics may develop, such as abnormal hair growth and deepening voice. Around menopause and after, many women notice increased growth of facial hair, and this may be due to an overbalance of male hormones.

MENSTRUATION AND MENOPAUSE

If you've stopped having periods, you may be relieved not to have to plan vacations around your "personal" schedule, or worry about "showing through" and having to carry your "supplies" with you. If you haven't stopped yet, you have these new freedoms to anticipate!

Menstruation and childbirth, as well as menopause, are natural aspects of the life cycle of women and are demonstrations of health, not illness.

Common Menstrual Problems of Midlife Women

There are some common, everyday menstrual problems that many midlife women experience. It helps to understand a little about the causes. There are some problems that you may want to treat yourself with self-help remedies. If problems persist or are severe, you should talk to your doctor about them.

Irregular periods

"I'm 52, 5'2", weigh 169 pounds, and still have unpredictable periods and such a heavy flow that I worry about "flooding." I've had some embarrassments while at work and am afraid of wearing light-colored clothing for fear that it will happen again. My doctor did a D and C and said "everything's normal," although I'm anemic and still am having hot flashes. I'm anxious for my menopause to finally happen and straighten me out."

"I am looking forward to menopause. I have had excessive bleeding for the past few years with my period."

"Why do I still have regular, extremely heavy periods at age 52? When will they stop?"

"I'm 49, 5'6", weigh 110 pounds, and exercise a lot. My periods have been lighter and lighter, although fairly regular, for about the last year. My doctor says I will probably stop menstruating soon."

Around menopause, periods take on many different patterns. They may be:

- Closer together
- Heavier or lighter
- Longer or shorter
- Gradually more spaced out
- Skipped for one or more months
- Skipped for even a year
- A skipped period followed by a longer, heavier period

HOW ESTROGEN LEVELS AFFECT MENSTRUATION There are many "normal" causes for irregular periods. One is an increase in estrogen and a decrease in progesterone. These ups and downs influence how your periods will change. Some obese women tend to have a great deal of estrogen, which might induce heavier periods, while the thin, athletic types may have less, accounting for a diminished flow and perhaps even earlier menopause.

The balance of these two hormones doesn't stay the same even in the same woman. During the premenopausal years, the level of estrogen may fall gradually, rapidly, or intermittently. Estrogen is responsible for building the lining of the uterus, and if the estrogen level is erratic, there will be erratic bleeding. A heavy supply of estrogen will cause frequent, continuous bleeding or very heavy bleeding.

HOW ANOVULATION AFFECTS MENSTRUATION Another normal cause of irregular periods is lack of ovulation. During a woman's forties, she may not ovulate, and without ovulation, predictable menstrual cycles do not occur. However, unpredictable bleeding can occur due to stimulation of the uterine lining from irregular hormone production. Sometimes doctors will prescribe progesterone, the "ovulation" hormone, to correct bleeding due to anovulation.

HOW UTERINE FIBROID TISSUE AFFECTS MENSTRUATION Many women have harmless "fibroids" or leiomas, which are hard, circular whorls of fibrous tissue, in their uterine muscle. This type of growth can occur at any age, but generally appears more frequently when women are in their forties because of high estrogen levels. Fibroids seem to grow under the influence of estrogens, so overweight women may be more prone to them.

Normally, the uterus contracts during a menstrual period, sometimes causing cramps. Fibroids may prevent this "clamping down" process, perhaps by increasing the surface area of the lining and preventing the muscle from contracting sufficiently. Therefore, women who have fibroids may have very long and/or heavy menses. These usually get a little better after menopause, without surgery.

HOW IUDs AFFECT MENSTRUATION IUD users usually bleed more during periods, possibly due to chronic inflammation of the uterine lining.

WHAT CAN YOU DO ABOUT IRREGULAR PERIODS? Keep a calendar. Make notes on a calendar to help you remember when your last period occurred and how long it lasted. Jot down other pertinent facts that you may want to discuss with your doctor, such as heavy flow or light flow.

You may find that what seems to you inexplicable bleeding actually falls into a new, but nonetheless predictable pattern (for you).

The following are "normal" patterns for some women:

- 21-day cycles
- Full menses every four weeks with midcycle spotting (some women interpret this pattern as periods every two weeks)
- 35 to 40-day cycles
- Monthly cycles with pre-, post-, and menstrual spotting

SELF-HELP FOR HEAVY BLEEDING After medical evaluation reveals that your heavy periods are not dangerous, these suggestions may make you feel better:

- *Take vitamins* Iron and B-Vitamin deficiency is the most common cause of anemia. Anemia can contribute to changes in menstrual patterns and interfere with your overall feeling of well-being. Extra iron and B vitamins will help your system cope with blood loss.
- *Reduce your estrogen level to help lighten a heavy flow* A drop in your estrogen level may contribute to changes in your menstrual patterns. Weight loss, an extremely low-fat diet, and regular exercise will help reduce your estrogen level and may even help relieve fibroids.
- *Be body conscious* Pay attention to your own signals. Chronic tiredness may be a tipoff that you are anemic. Pain might be a warning that you have an infection. Watch for signs of pregnancy, particularly if you are an IUD user. Remember to have a Pap smear performed once a year.

CAUSES OF BLEEDING TO BE CONCERNED ABOUT Don't let minor changes in menstrual patterns worry you. For example, IUDs can make periods heavier. For some women, birth control pills keep periods light. Some women may notice an increase in flow after cessation of birth control pills.

While some women who have had tubal ligations report an increase in menstrual flow, it is at present unclear whether tubal ligation aggravates bleeding or whether women simply happen to have tubals at a time when they are likely to have irregular bleeding anyway.

When menstrual periods begin to change, there is an increasing chance of development of uterine fibroids.

There are several less common but more serious reasons for irregular periods.

Several types of cancers can cause spotting or irregular bleeding:

- Cervix (detected by Pap test)
- Uterus (not detected by Pap test), can be detected by D and C or uterine biopsy
- Ovarian cancer, which may stimulate estrogen secretion, which in turn overstimulates the uterine lining (detected either by pelvic exam or ultrasound)

Uterine infections will interfere with regular menses, especially with IUD use.

Additionally, the following benign/precancerous conditions will interfere with menses:

- Endometrial hyperplasia: An overgrowth of the uterine lining. Some types of hyperplasia are considered precancerous; others are not.
- Polyps in the cervix or uterine lining.
- Ovarian cysts. These will interrupt the menstrual cycle. Since some ovarian cysts are malignant, enlarged ovaries must be evaluated by examinations and, at times, ultrasound or even surgical removal.

SUMMING UP: HEAVY/IRREGULAR PERIODS Heavy or irregular periods are the norm for women in their late thirties through early fifties. Since there are a few dangerous causes of bleeding in addition to many less serious ones, this is an important time of your life to have regular gynecologic checkups. It will help to keep a careful menstrual calendar of bleeding days and spotting days. This helps to tell whether your bleeding is truly unpredictable or simply falls into a different pattern than you are accustomed to. But in addition to keeping a calendar and reporting annually for checkups, there are certain times that you should seek medical attention *immediately*. They include:

- Hemorrhage.
- Continual spotting, especially if using an IUD.
- Continual spotting, expecially if accompanied by pain.
- Continual spotting, especially if you could be pregnant. Spotting could be a sign of a serious infection or tubal pregnancy.
- Any bleeding pattern that is accompanied by severe pain, high temperature, or a feeling of being very ill.

Premenstrual syndrome (PMS)

A second major area of complaints of midlife women is premenstrual syndrome. Premenstrual syndrome (PMS) is the name given to a group of symptoms experienced during the two weeks prior to menses and occasionally at midcycle.

For many women, premenstrual syndrome may include:

- Irritability and mood changes
- Bloating and fluid retention
- Breast tenderness
- Headache
- Food cravings (for example, for sugary foods)
- Depression

Many women have some common complaints during the days before menstruation begins, but only about two to three percent of all women develop severely disabling symptoms.

The symptoms that some of the currently menopausal generation have experienced for 30 years now have a medical name. In the last decade, PMS has become a recognized syndrome, although premenstrual tension and other problems have been described by women for many years. PMS seems most commonly to affect women in their late thirties and forties who have had children, although younger women have it, too. This group may be different hormonally from women who have not had children and younger women. Additionally, since many young mothers today often are chronically exhausted and under enormous stress due to conflicting demands of career and family, this group may simply have lower physical and emotional reserves for coping with problems. Stress and fatigue may exacerbate their physical symptoms.

There are several possible causes of PMS. These may vary among women because hormonal levels differ so much. All or some of the following may relate to PMS:

- Imbalance between estrogen/progesterone levels.
- Fluid retention, which may affect the central nervous system.
- A defect in the central nervous system neurotransmitter regulation. The dopamine* system is most commonly suspected, since this affects mood, and disruptions in the dopaminergic system relate to mood swings and depression.
- A related pituitary hormone, prolactin, has been suspected as a cause of PMS. In humans, prolactin is involved in production of breast milk. Interestingly, in fish, prolactin is involved in fluid metabolism. Perhaps this function occurs in humans also, and explains why women with PMS so commonly complain of bloating and fluid retention.

HELPING YOURSELF WITH PMS Keep a record of your symptoms. You'll probably find that they fall into a pattern. Some PMS sufferers commonly say they feel that they are losing their minds because they think their symptoms are occurring unpredictably. Simply discovering the pattern may make the symptoms more manageable.

Rest When you have some idea of when PMS symptoms are likely to occur, simply getting extra rest can help.

Diet Dietary changes can also help. Several foods seem to aggravate PMS. These include caffeine and other stimulants, sugars, sweets, and processed, artificial foods that may contain a high proportion of sugar, salt, and some spices. A low-salt, low-sugar diet with lots of fiber and frequent small meals may help PMS sufferers.

Exercise Exercise may contribute to your general feeling of well-being and reduce fluid retention. Also, exercise may release endorphins into the system and help undo the disruption going on in your dopamine system.

Vitamins Vitamins, particulary B_6, C, and E, have been used to relieve PMS symptoms for many women. You may want to try them. Buy small

---

*Dopamine. The dopaminergic system is a system of neurotransmitters that seems to be involved with our hormonal metabolism, changing our moods, and causing depression. Hormones, antidepressants, and narcotics all interact with the dopaminergic system, although the exact mechanisms are not well understood.

quantities, start taking them in small doses, and see if you notice any difference in how you feel.

Support groups Support groups at women's health centers may be helpful.

WHEN TO SEEK MEDICAL HELP FOR PMS

- When you've tried the suggestions listed above and they haven't worked for you
- When your symptoms are so severe that they are causing family /marital/work problems
- When your symptoms make you feel violent or suicidal

THERAPIES FOR PMS

"You're not unique. Irritating as it is, try a few of the alternatives and it's not a problem. The first offered alternative may not be your solution."

There are medications to help women who have clinically significant difficulties as part of PMS. Current therapies for PMS include:

- Hormones
- Vitamins, especially B$_6$ supplements
- Tranquilizers
- Antidepressants
- Herbal remedies

While some women benefit from Vitamin B$_6$ supplements (pyroxidine), these should be used with caution because overdoses have been known to cause nerve damage.

Progesterone is most frequently used to treat PMS hormonally. It has been used in the form of injections, vaginal and rectal suppositories, or pills. There are advantages and disadvantages to each form. While the efficacy of progesterone for PMS treatment has not been proven, many women believe it helps dramatically, and it does not seem to have any dangerous risks. Some women improve on birth control pills, but long-term use of birth control pills is not recommended after age 40.

For most women, loss of weight, careful attention to a well-balanced diet, reduction of salt intake, additional rest and relaxation, long walks, or warm baths may relieve symptoms of PMS. You may not have to resort to medications that may have unpleasant side effects. Sedatives and tranquilizers have been tried, but in general they are not very useful for PMS.

VAGINAL DRYNESS—THE PROBLEM NO ONE TALKS ABOUT

"The vaginal dryness bothers me the most."

"I thought I was the only one who had a dry vagina. I didn't know that vaginal dryness bothered other women until I received your questionnaire and then told a few friends about the questions. They said they had this problem, too, and that started a whole discussion."

Here's a topic many women don't even discuss with each other! In our survey, 36.7% of the respondents said vaginal dryness was a problem. (Some of the men in their lives are concerned about it, too!) What happens to the vaginal tract and why does dryness present difficulties?

The major problems are:

- Chronic discomfort of itching and irritation
- Tendency to repeated vaginal infections
- Discomfort during sexual intercourse

Estrogen deficiency causes the vagina to become shorter and less elastic. Decreasing blood supply causes the vaginal mucosa to become pale, and the vaginal tissues to become increasingly fragile and susceptible to infection. (More about vaginal infections and how to treat them in chapter 10.)

Many women have noticed that, as their vaginal tract becomes drier, sexual intercourse becomes uncomfortable, even painful. For those with a seriously dry condition, irritation and bleeding may result. Needless to say, interest in sexual activity may diminish rapidly under these circumstances. Many women do not understand what is happening inside their bodies at this time, and some wonder if they are not sufficiently stimulated by their husband or lover.

Overcoming Vaginal Dryness and Urinary Tract Difficulties

Around the time of menopause, reduced supplies of estrogen may cause the walls of your vagina to become less elastic, thinner, and drier, making the vagina more vulnerable to infection. Many women become more susceptible to urinary tract infections as the tissues in the genital area change. Also, stress incontinence—losing a little urine while laughing, coughing, or exercising—happens to some women.

Everyday help for vaginal dryness

- Avoid irritating, drying soaps, bubble bath preparations, and fragranced items in your bath water.

- Wear loose-fitting clothing around your crotch. Panties with cotton crotch panels are best for avoiding irritation.
- If you must be girdled/pantyhosed all day long, put on a free-flowing T-shirt, robe, or nightgown in the evening without any panties. (If you have a mate or lover, this attire may interest him, too!)
- In general, douching is unnecessary and can cause drying, irritating effects. However, occasional mild vinegar or Betadine douches may head off infections in early stages.
- Some women swear by yogurt, and even douche with it on the theory that it makes vaginal secretions more resistant to infection. (The authors suggest that if you try this, use plain yogurt.) (See chapter 10 for other recommendations from the Federation of Feminist Health Centers.)
- Estrogen cream inserted vaginally may improve the tone of the vaginal walls. You can use a lower dose with vaginally administered estrogen than with orally administered estrogen.
- Adequate foreplay prior to intercourse will increase vaginal secretions.
- Frequent intercourse seems to stimulate the vaginal walls and keep them stronger.

Vaginal Dryness and Surgery

Another reason for vaginal dryness is the aftereffect of surgery. Those who have had hysterectomies may find that some of their mucus secreting glands have been destroyed. Vaginal dryness makes intercourse difficult. However, most women still can have adequate vaginal lubrication even after surgery. The same self-help suggestions given above apply to post-hysterectomy vaginal dryness.

Vaginal Dryness and Sexual Activity

To combat dryness and to make sexual intercourse a pleasanter experience, use about a teaspoonful of water-soluble jelly, such as K-Y, on the outside of your vagina. You might also put a little inside. Your mate may help you apply it as part of foreplay. The lubricant will mix with your own natural lubrication and enhance nature's contributions.

Keep in mind that vaginal dryness is reversible. Even if you have not had sexual intercourse for a long time, your lubrication will probably return with appropriate interest and stimulation.

INCONTINENCE: NO ONE EVER DIED FROM LEAKING URINE

Many women around age 50 and after find themselves running to the women's room oftener than they did when they were younger. More importantly, many find that they lose a little urine when laughing, coughing, or perhaps during exercise such as jogging or aerobic dancing.

Perhaps nearly half of women over age 50 have various bladder complaints. In our survey, 48.5% of the respondents reported loss of urine.

In the past, many women may not have complained about this problem. They may have felt embarrassment, or that it was something that they would have to live with. Now, women have greater expectations regarding their health and physical capabilities and discuss these problems with their doctors. Until recently, doctors were not very concerned about this problem. No one ever died from leaking urine!

In some women urinary leakage is caused by the effects of childbirth. In others, recurring bladder infections or nervous bladder instability lead to urinary leakage. With decreasing estrogen levels, some sagging of the bladder support structures occurs.

Childbearing and sexual activity stretch the vaginal opening and make it hard to tighten vaginal muscles that also control release of urine. Excessive "pushing down" from other causes—such as obesity, chronic coughing, chronic constipation, and possibly regular jogging—may aggravate an already-weak bladder.

Irritable bladder can result from overuse of stimulants such as caffeine, nicotine, diet pills, amphetamines, and asthma medications. Avoid caffeine and smoking, and take only necessary medications. Typical symptoms of urinary frequency or urgency (having to "run" once the urge strikes) are a chronic sense of "having to go" and urinating only small amounts. Urinary tract infections can cause bladder irritation, so if symptoms occur suddenly, seek medical attention.

Diabetes can cause incontinence, as can some serious illnesses, such as multiple sclerosis and spinal cord tumors.

What to Do

One way to strengthen the muscles that control the flow of urine is by doing exercises known as Kegels (named for Dr. A. M. Kegel). These exercises have helped many women with bladder control. They can also contribute to the overall tone of your pelvic area.

You can begin the exercises with three short sessions each day and gradually work up to three longer sessions. Here's what to do:

1. Become aware of your PC (pubucoccygeus) muscles. They surround your vagina and anus, forming a kind of double "sling,"

starting at the pubic bone and looping under the vagina and anus. How to know which muscles: When you insert a tampon, you can squeeze it with these muscles. When you stop the flow of urine in midstream, these are the muscles you use. Also, you know the sensation of "holding back" on a bowel movement. That's the same set of muscles.

2. Begin by contracting the muscles about 25 times per session, three sessions each day.

3. Work up to three sessions of 100 or more contractions. You can do these exercises while seated at your desk, watching TV, riding on a bus, and even while making love!

Being aware of how you can contract and relax these muscles may also contribute to your sexual enjoyment. Your ability to squeeze these muscles around your partner's erect penis may give you and your partner added dimensions of pleasure and may help you achieve orgasm. (Some writers have referred to the PC as the "love muscles.")

Other ways to prevent loss of urine

- Lose weight
- Avoid stimulants mentioned above
- If the problem is really disruptive to your life, surgery can help
- To avoid constipation, eat a high-fiber diet and drink plenty of liquids

Your doctor will test you for possible disease, urinary tract infection, and nerve disorders. You may also have studies of your bladder capacity and function and X-ray studies of your bladder and kidney. For a discussion of severe urinary incontinence, see chapter 3.

BREASTS

Our breasts seem to cause many of us concern at all ages. After middle age, many women notice:

- Breast size diminishes
- With excessive weight gain, breast size may increase
- Breasts may flatten or droop

During and after menopause, the shape and size of breasts may change somewhat. A steady supply of estrogen influences the glandular, fibrous, and fatty tissues that make up the breasts. After menopause, the breasts may diminish slightly in size, as fatty tissue is replaced by fibrous tissue. The skin of the breast does not shrink at the same rate as the underlying tissue, giving the breasts of thin women a flattened appearance and those of obese women a "drooping" appearance. Regardless of body shape and size, the nipples may become smaller and flatter and lose their erectile properties.

Many women worry unnecessarily about changes in their breasts, since many of us (wrongly) assume everybody else looks like *Playboy* bunnies (even the bunnies don't look like that when the underwiring, silicone, and photographic touchups are removed!) Size and shape are really unimportant; sexual responsiveness usually relates to how a woman feels about her body, whatever nature gave her!

A well-fitted bra can help your appearance in clothes. Good breast support throughout your life is important to overcome the "drooping" appearance that can develop over time; after menopause adequate support is even more important. You may want to consider changing bra styles if you've been wearing the same style for a number of years.

While exercises won't help increase your dimensions (despite what the ads in the women's magazines say), exercise will help firm up the muscles in your chest and upper arms. With good muscle tone, your overall appearance will be better.

(You'll read more about medical problems associated with breasts in chapter 3.)

Fibrocystic Breasts

Painful, lumpy breasts are a common complaint. So-called "fibrocystic disease" affects a large percentage of women. Fortunately, several simple measures may improve this condition. A research study at Johns Hopkins University showed that cysts were eliminated in 80% of women who changed their lifestyles, says Marvin Posner, M.D., medical director of one of Empire HMO's groups, the Community Health Plan of Suffolk, Hauppauge, New York, and Associate Professor, Department of Community and Preventive Medicine, State University of New York at Stony Brook. "Women who have cystic mastitis should avoid caffeine, chocolate products, give up smoking, and take 800 international units of Vitamin E each day. Research is under way to understand the precise mechanism of why and how Vitamin E is effective in this situation." (More about fibrocystic breasts in the next chapter.)

WEIGHT GAIN

As time changes, your body rearranges. This could be the theme song of middle age! Around menopause (and even before), many women notice slight changes in their shapes. Few look as they did at age 25. Body fat redistributes.

Many notice bulges around the abdomen, despite efforts to exercise and stay fit. In some, this may be due to actual increase in fat, while in others it is due to a change in metabolism of fat.

Many women fight the aging process with exercise, diet, and even plastic surgery. Others prefer to accept the inevitable gracefully, while maintaining their levels of energy, health, and vitality.

For many women, weight gain is one of the most dreaded of changes of the climacteric and the most misunderstood. It is *not* inevitable, but is caused by changing activity, changing metabolism, and changing hormones.

Where has your weight gone? Up, down, all around? Here's what happens to some women:

- "Estrogenized" women tend to put weight on the hips and thighs.
- Perimenopausal women tend to put on weight around the waistline.
- Many women notice that their metabolism is slower and that their weight goes up even though they eat the same amount that they did before.
- A lucky few get an increased metabolic rate from androgens and either lose a little weight or maintain their weight. Androgens tend to increase muscle mass, and muscle has a higher metabolic rate (burns calories faster) than fat.

In the Holt-Kahn survey, 15.2% of the women reported a more-than-30-pound weight gain; 41.4% reported a mild weight gain; 43.3% no weight gain.

What to Do About an "Expanding" Body Shape

Fight weight gain! Diet and exercise! This is a good time to gain a new lease on your body. Your career may be slowing down and the demands of child rearing may have lightened. It's time to take care of yourself. You can't afford not to!

Also, it's time to think about what you really want to be: Try to feel good about yourself rather than a slave to how you think you "should be." First, choose a target weight that is realistic and comfortable for you. Your own "ideal" weight may be a few pounds more or less than the "ideal" found in charts. Recognize that a healthy, fit, happy woman who is 10 pounds over "ideal" is better off than a woman who is constantly on a seesaw of fad diets and obsessed with losing that 10 pounds.

Having picked a suitable weight, you should then find a balance of exercise and food intake to maintain it. Low-calorie diets will result in weight loss, but unless you exercise vigorously your metabolic rate may also slow down. Also, midlife women often complain of "flab" even when they get to a good weight. Poor muscle tone leads to midriff bulge unless you also exercise. The take-home messages of this section are:

- Be realistic about your weight
- Like yourself (You needn't look like Sophia Loren or Lena Horne or Jackie Onassis to be healthy, happy, and attractive.)
- Exercise
- Eat moderately (You'll read more about nutrition in chapter 8.)

SKIN AND HAIR CHANGES

As we age, we notice changes in our skin before many other physical changes. We often guess our friends' and acquaintances' ages by these visible signs. "Changes in the skin, such as loss of elasticity, color, thickness and moisture, echo changes elsewhere in the body," says Arthur K. Balin, M.D., Ph.D., Assistant Professor and Associate Physician at The Rockefeller University Hospital in New York City.

In general, as we age, skin loses some tone and gets drier, moles may darken, "sun spots" may appear, little pin-head-size red splotches may appear, and varicose veins may become more prominent.

Skin "tags" may develop. Skin tags are mole-like appendages, extra pieces of skin that hang, usually from armpit or neck. Skin tags do not become cancerous, but they can become irritated and even bleed. Skin tags seem to be due to an increasing tendency of aging skin to lay down melanin, the dark pigment most noticeable in moles. Moles also normally enlarge at midlife, but large moles *can* become malignant and should be assessed by a physician.

Our skin, our largest and most accessible organ, changes in response to diminished levels of estrogen. The major changes seem to be thinning and drying, resulting in creases and lines, an increased tendency toward itching, and slight thinning of hair. The high estrogen level in young women is responsible, in large part, for their good skin tone and moisture retention. However, high levels of estrogen can also lead to edema and bloating.

What to Do About Skin Changes, Wrinkles, and Age Spots

Avoid weight fluctuations. Fluctuations alternatively fill out and reduce tissue mass, leading to wrinkling.

Avoid excessive sun exposure. Prevent sunburn by using a sunscreen if you must be in the sun for a long period. This will reduce the darkening of freckles and moles and the appearance of skin tags and "age spots." Sun also damages the skin and aggravates wrinkling.

Don't smoke. Smoking increases wrinkling and isn't attractive.

Use nondrying soaps. If you want to use soap on your face, pure glycerine soap is less drying than others. Some cosmetologists advise using other cleansing preparations on the face, such as specially formulated milk baths. Use moisturizers liberally.

Deal with separate areas of your face and neck in separate ways. For example, you may have oily areas around your nose and on your chin. You may want to protect areas prone to wrinkling, such as around your eyelids, under your eyes, and your neck, by using different cleansing agents there.

Some women get an increase in acne from male hormones. This can be treated locally with careful washing and over-the-counter benzoil peroxide agents. In severe cases a physician might suggest other medications.

What About Hair Changes?

How much facial and body hair a woman has depends on her heredity, her male and female hormone levels, and the sensitivity of hormone "receptors" in the skin. Hormonal levels are affected by ovarian and adrenal hormone production as well as interconversion of hormones in skin and fatty tissues. Needless to say, there are many reasons why hair growth patterns change at midlife, when all of the glandular functions may be changing!

One common midlife change is generalized thinning of hair. This is a "female" pattern due to decreasing estrogen levels. It can be minimized by general good physical care and good hair conditioning and styling. There is no simple treatment for this pattern baldness. A doctor will check for diseases that can cause hair loss. A local cream (minoxidil) is being tested for "male pattern" baldness but its safety is unclear and its role in "female pattern" baldness is unclear. Some women note improvement with estrogen replacement.

Another common midlife change is increasing facial and body hair. This is related to several changes: a slight increase in adrenal androgens as ovarian hormone production declines; or the effects of circulating androgens may be more noticeable. Obese women have higher levels of both estrogens and androgens and a higher rate of anovulation; hence male pattern hair growth (hirsutism) seems more common in obese women.

Alternatives for treatment of hair growth include simply plucking, or waxing or electrolysis. Plucking and waxing remove the hairs; they neither help nor hurt the growth. Electrolysis destroys the hair follicle.

There is also a medication originally used only as a diuretic that has been reported to block androgen effects in the skin and to decrease hirsutism. Although this medication (spironolactone) is not approved by the FDA for this use and its effects are gradual and subtle, many women find it helpful. One gynecologist commented that although women complained that the spironolactone was not very effective, they almost all refused to stop using it, making it seem that it must be more helpful than they would admit! Spironolactone is a diuretic and has potential side effects, but its use to date has been free of catastrophic problems. A similar drug called cytoproterone acetate is used in other countries for hirsutism.

What to do about hair changes

Occasionally hirsutism can be caused by ovarian or adrenal tumors. Most women, however, have hormone levels in the normal range and either skin receptors that are supersensitive to normal hormonal levels or an unrealistic idea of how much facial and body hair a woman of their age, weight, and ethnic background should have. Women from Mediterranean backgrounds typically have more hair. Very fair women may not be aware of hair changes, since their fairer hair may not be as noticeable. Conversely, fair women may be accustomed to little facial or body hair and react very strongly to midlife changes. We offer the following suggestions:

- You can help the condition of your hair by staying well nourished. Hair responds to general body health. If you feel run down and do not have as much energy as you think you should have, multivitamins may help you feel better and also help the condition of your hair. Also, consider having a permanent wave or a new hair style, or wearing a hairpiece or wig.
- If you notice a sudden change in your hair, tell your doctor. Remember, hair follicles take six months to change. Major stress or hormonal changes may propel all hair follicles into an involutional stage together, leading to myths about hair falling out. Hair loss is normally a continuous process, but in healthy women, new hair constantly replaces the old.
- You can also shape your eyebrows and pluck stray hairs that appear around your face and neck.
- If you have excessive facial hair on your upper lip, you might want to bleach it or use wax to remove it. Also, you might consider electrolysis, which destroys individual follicles but does not keep new ones from forming.
- If you don't like gray hair, change it. Hair colorings are available in temporary rinses that wash out and more permanent dyes that "grow" out. Only your hairdresser need know for sure! Colorings and permanents also increase the fullness or body of hair, which can counteract the gradual thinning resulting from falling estrogen levels.

- Be content with some imperfections. Blemishes are more noticeable to some women than to others. Remember that the American cultural norm of what is attractive is generally based on the fair, light-skinned Northern European look. Women from southern cultures almost always have more body hair. Rarely do men seem bothered by body hair. It is usually women who are much more conscious of "excess" hair after poring over magazine pictures of models (who probably shave and pluck and have the photos touched up to achieve that hairless, smooth look).

VARICOSE VEINS

Varicose veins on the legs seem to be more noticeable as women age. Often a tendency to have varicose veins is hereditary. If your mother or grandmother had them, you may also have them. Varicose veins also occur in individuals who have nutritional deficiencies and who consume large amounts of alcohol. Smoking may also aggravate varicose veins. Don't smoke.

Varicose veins usually are not uncomfortable, but in more advanced cases aching can occur. Dangerous blood clots and thrombophlebitis are related to the deeper veins, not the superficial ones that are visible.

"Women who have a hereditary tendency to varicose veins should be careful not to augment that tendency," says Dr. Posner. He gives the following self-help suggestions:

- Exercise enough so that you use your legs and encourage better circulation throughout your body.
- Be aware that crossing your legs for prolonged periods of time can interfere with blood circulation.
- Avoid wearing tight garters (does anyone, anymore?) and tying stockings up on the thigh in a knot (the way some of our grandmothers did).
- Wear support hose. They are now available in very fashionable styles and colors.
- Avoid prolonged standing or sitting in one position.
- If you have varicose veins, sit with your legs elevated whenever possible.
- Don't smoke.

Additional suggestions from the authors:

- Keep your weight down.
- Space your pregnancies (a little late to tell you now); several closely spaced pregnancies can aggravate or cause varicose veins.

If a doctor suggests a surgical procedure, ask if it is *medically* necessary or if it is being suggested solely for cosmetic purposes. While many women are sensitive about their veins, many others are willing to live with a painless situation that just doesn't look as pretty as clear-skinned legs. Surgical procedures *do* carry risks, and surgery should be avoided unless it is necessary.

In severe cases, surgical stripping can be performed. Also, there is an injection treatment, in which trapped blood is forced out and replaced by a salt solution, and the discolored vein segment collapses and is absorbed. In some women, tiny purple veins may reappear.

YOUR EYES: CAN YOU STILL THREAD A NEEDLE?

"My arm isn't long enough for me to read the newspaper or a menu in a restaurant. When I asked my date to hold the menu across the table for me to read, I knew I needed reading glasses."

Visual changes often occur in women, as well as men, after age 40 or 45. If you have worn glasses for many years, you may notice that you need to change your prescription more often. You may have to take off your glasses when you want to read something up close. If you never needed glasses before, you may find that you need them now to thread a needle, read the newspaper, and see small objects clearly.

Statistically, presbyopia (inability to see at close range) occurs between the ages of 35 and 50. The lens of our eye, which focuses light on the retina, is held by a series of muscles that contract or relax to enable the lens to flatten or thicken to focus on distant or close objects. We see things well at a distance when the lens is thin. We see things far away when the lens is thick. As we age, there is less protein available to induce the lens to accommodate, and that is when we begin to experience uncomfortable near vision.

Fortunately, glasses now can be a high fashion item, and some of the world's most glamorous women are featured in eyeglass advertisements. Or, for many, wearing contact lenses is the answer.

SLEEP DIFFICULTIES

Many women experience changes in their sleep patterns around menopause. Some changes may be due to hot flashes or to many other factors involving stress.

Some changes are normal and should not cause alarm, according to Dudley Dinner, M.D., Director, Sleep Disorders Center, The Cleveland Clinic

Foundation. Although you may have slept seven to eight hours at age 20, you may need only six to six-and-a-half hours of sleep between ages 55 and 60. Also, your sleep may appear to become more "fragmented." You may awaken more often and spend more time awake during the night. Your total time in bed may increase.

The most frequently reported sleep problems relate to two categories. One is disorders of initiating or maintaining sleep (DIMS). These include:

- Difficulty getting to sleep
- Difficulty staying asleep
- Waking too early

The other category is disorders of excessive sleepiness (DOES). Complaints may include:

- Excessive daytime sleepiness
- Falling asleep inappropriately

Inadequate sleep may be the cause of this complaint, but other, more serious sleep disturbances may include:

- *Sleep apnea* This involves brief periods of ceasing to breathe. Some people cease breathing so often during the night and rouse themselves so often that they are tired all day and are likely to drift off to sleep at any moment. They are snorers, often overweight, and have elevated blood pressure, says Dr. Dinner.
- *Repetitive nocturnal myclonus* This consists of involuntary jerking movements of the legs, which disturb sleep. "Restless legs" refers to an uncomfortable sensation that occurs just before falling asleep. The individual feels an urge to get up and walk around. This sensation may increase with age and frequently runs in families, according to some researchers. It is more common in individuals aged 50 to 60 than in younger people.
- *Sleep disturbances related to medication* Some drugs, such as propranolol, cause sleepiness. Many midlife people take sleeping pills under a physician's prescription, which may make sleep apnea worse.
- *Sleep disturbances related to psychiatric factors* The major disturbance is clinical depression. (You'll read more about this in chapter 9.)

Understanding Sleep

Understanding the natural sleep cycle may help you cope better with your sleep disturbances. Sleep consists of a series of stages that occur in regular order in about 90-minute cycles. The cycle occurs four or five times during the night and influences alertness during waking hours.

A sleep cycle means uninterrupted sleep. For many women whose hot flashes awaken them, sleep cycles are disturbed. Such women may complain of frequent insomnia as well as irritability, depression, and reduced memory. Experimental sleep deprivation has been known to cause memory impairment, and menopausal women's complaints about memory may be related to a loss of REM sleep, the stage at the end of the sleep cycle.

How to Get a Good Night's Sleep

Most women say it takes them an average of about 15 minutes to go to sleep. Getting there may not be "as easy as falling off a log" for some individuals. If you have trouble getting to sleep and staying asleep long enough to feel energetic throughout the day, here are some suggestions. Some may be old ideas to you, but it may be time to try them again!

- Drink a cup of warm milk before bedtime. Eat a light snack. Avoid stimulating beverages that contain caffeine, such as coffee, tea, cola, and chocolate.
- Take a warm, relaxing bath. Use bubbles or an appealing fragrance (unless, of course, you are avoiding bubble baths due to vaginal or skin irritation or dryness). Take your time. Don't hurry. Luxuriate.
- Relax in bed and read something you enjoy. As your mind becomes engrossed, your muscles will relax. When your body is relaxed, you are likelier to become sleepy. Watching television may have the same effect. The programs or reading should be mildly enjoyable, but not scary or stimulating.
- Or read something you find very dull. When your mind can't handle what you present, your internal coping mechanism of falling asleep may take over.
- Experiment with changes in your environment. Is your bedroom too warm? Too cold? Do you sleep better with a window slightly open? Use different combinations of covers. Do you sleep better with a feeling of the weight of the blankets? If you like warmth without weight, try an electric blanket. Many have dual controls so that each bedpartner can choose his or her own level of heat.
- Avoid stressful situations before bedtime. Postpone discussions of problems until morning, whenever possible. Avoid lengthy

telephone conversations that may stimulate or upset you before bedtime.

- If you have an argument or tension-filled discussion late at night, don't go to bed mad. If the object of your anger is your bed mate, try to kiss and make up before sleep time.
- If you are alone and feeling upset, call a friend and talk. Venting may help you unload and sleep much better. (Women who live alone need a friend to call at such times.)
- "Avoid using sleeping pills. People build up a tolerance to them. Pills have daytime hypnotic effects. And flurazepam induces sleep apnea in some cases," warns Donald Bliwise, Ph.D., of the Sleep Disorders Center, Stanford University Medical School. "There are few good indications for using sleeping pills," says Dr. Bliwise. "A doctor or pharmacist can describe the different kinds of sleeping pills available. Nightly use of any hypnotic won't be effective after a while. We encourage use (if they have to be used at all), only once every third night. We find people who use alcohol to help sleeping pills work after they have built up a tolerance to the sleeping pills. Some combine alcohol and sleeping pills unconsciously. Heavy drinking plus pills leads to big tolerance for both, and neither works after a while."
- "We do not recommend napping during the day. One half-hour of sleep during the day can affect sleep at night."
- "If you have trouble going to sleep, stay up late until you feel yourself becoming drowsy. Only at that point should you go into the bedroom and lie down," recommends Dr. Bliwise.
- Hugs, kisses, and sexual activity may promote sound sleep.
- If a mate's snoring bothers you, try using wax ear plugs. And have your mate get a medical checkup. "The snorer should let his/her partner go to sleep first," says Dr. Posner.

If you want 342 pages of suggestions for getting better sleep, read The American Medical Association's book, *Straight Talk, No-Nonsense Guide to Better Sleep.* You'll find more details on many of the topics outlined in this chapter and much more, including a directory of Sleep Disorder Centers to help you locate an expert in case you need professional help in getting that all-important sleep.

The Morning After

If you have a sleepless night, get up and keep active all throughout the next day, advises Dr. Cartwright. "Run around the block, jump rope, or do something physically active to oxygenate your body. You will feel less tired all day long and the activity will help you sleep better that night. I don't recommend taking a nap during the day to compensate for the lost sleep."

NONSPECIFIC CHANGES

During the climacteric, there are many nonspecific changes, both physical and mental.

After menopause, because of the aging process, women are at somewhat increased risk for organic disease. Don't let your doctor write off chest pains, headache, and other symptoms just as part of menopause. These symptoms should be investigated to rule out more serious conditions that require more specific treatment.

Sometimes there are changes in the function of the thyroid gland after menopause. Hypothyroidism may "slow down" the body, leading to weight gain and mental and physical lethargy. Hyperthyroidism may bring on sweating, rapid heart beat, nervousness, and temperature instability. Separating thyroid symptoms from changes in the circulatory system associated with menopause requires careful attention and thorough investigation by your physician.

> *"I always thought a lot of the midlife problems were in the mind, until I got here. Now I think they're very real."*

> *"Any woman who thinks menopause is going to be traumatic will dwell on the problems of it and that increases the problems."*

PSYCHOLOGICAL CHANGES

> *"If your doctor tells you menopausal problems are 'all in your mind,' go to another doctor!"*

The old saying "It's all in your head," does apply to some of the changes of menopause. Many women describe irritability, depression, a feeling that they just can't cope, sleeplessness, and lack of energy, and most women do experience some psychological changes around the time of menopause. There is uncertainty about the hormonal and psychological basis for these complaints.

In previous generations, women regarded themselves as "deteriorating" when their reproductive years were over. They thought of themselves as sexually less attractive than younger women, and these feelings led to some degree of depression. Even now, hot flashes during a business meeting or vaginal discomfort during intercourse can contribute to emotional as well as practical problems.

But now, with the combination of changes in lifestyle and medical therapy, many women can overcome the problems of depression whether the cause is related to stress or stems from physical problems. Medical problems associated with physical changes due to the aging process can be dealt with by a variety of medical specialists. The important thing to remember is that many problems are preventable—or even reversible. And there are many things you can do to help yourself. For example, exercise more. Exercise usually gives most women a sense of well-being. And, remember, the "empty nest syndrome" only affects "nesting" women!

Many women report rapid mood swings, from high to low, or from low to high. Many report periods of ongoing depression. Whether these conditions are due to the physical changes brought about by the hormonal changes within the body or by extraneous psychosocial factors should be analysed for each individual. There are many psychosocial factors that midlife women encounter that may influence their mental attitudes and abilities to cope with physical and mental changes. You'll read more about them in chapter 9.

3
WHEN MEDICAL HELP
IS NECESSARY

Although self-help can overcome many problems as we saw in chapter 2, unfortunately, there are times when a woman must depend upon the medical system. Indeed, failure to do so may cost her life.

In this chapter you'll read about some of the more serious women's midlife health problems and what is commonly done about them. It would take a medical encyclopedia to list them all, so this discussion will be limited to questions that respondents to our survey have raised: disorders of the uterus, endometriosis, pelvic inflammatory disease, disorders of the ovaries, breast disease, breast surgery, and urinary tract problems. You'll also read about mammography and breast reconstruction after mastectomy.

Most of the serious health problems affecting midlife women are surrounded by controversies over treatment. Controversies are confusing to the professional and even more so to the layperson. Be aware of the treatment alternatives and find a doctor whom you trust and with whom you feel comfortable. Also consider seeking a second opinion before any treatment is initiated.

> "Too many male doctors are still inclined to brush off menopause complaints as minor problems that you should learn to live with, then they get all shook up because of a cancerous endometrium."

> "It is not a period in your life you have to be afraid about; just be informed with the correct facts about it and ask your doctor any questions."

Many women who responded to our questionnaire commented about difficulties in finding a sympathetic doctor. Such doctors are out there —keep looking! There are also referral services offered by several health organizations and self-help groups. However, be sure your doctor is doing what is medically appropriate, since the best bedside manner in the world will not make up for poor medical care.

Many "women's" books imply an adversarial relationship between woman and doctor. This is unfortunate, since a critical attitude may put a doctor on the defensive and result in poor communications.

You have a right to expect courtesy, kindness, and honesty from your doctor; you should feel that he or she is taking enough time to answer your questions and is not unduly pressuring you into a treatment that you do not want. However, in return, recognize that doctors are human beings who also respond best to courteous behavior. Recognize that your doctor may often be tired and pressed for time. Do everyone a favor and have your questions and concerns clearly in mind. This chapter will help you do that. And you'll find some suggestions for understanding why doctors are the way they are and how to get along better with them in the future in chapter 11.

In this chapter you'll read a little bit about a lot of things, ranging from screening procedures, such as the Pap smear, to serious medical problems. Knowing more will help you make your lists of questions when you go for checkups and visits to specialists.

THE PAP SMEAR

Most gynecologists recommend that at midlife you have a yearly pelvic examination, including a Pap smear. This is a scraping of cells from the cervix. It is 95% accurate for detecting cervical cancer, and occasionally a uterine cancer will be detected from it.

Fortunately, a common abnormality named "dysplasia," or cervical intraepithelial neoplasia (CIN), usually predates cancer by several years. Dysplasia often improves after treatment with antibiotics, freezing, or laser surgery, so the woman who has regular Pap smears can be treated for dysplasia and will probably never develop cervical cancer. Once cancer has occurred, hysterectomy and/or radiation treatments may be necessary.

Pap smears are "graded" from I (normal) to IV or V (cancer). Labs differ in how serious a class II or III may be, but any smear other than I should be discussed with your doctor.

After a hysterectomy, the cervix is gone, so in general, Pap smears are not nearly as important. However, if a hysterectomy was done for cervical or uterine cancer, regular Pap smears should continue since the vaginal "cuff" is the most common recurrence site. In addition, many doctors continue to recommend Pap smears since the test is fairly inexpensive and can be useful in detecting vaginal abnormalities, hormonal changes, and some forms of sexually transmitted diseases.

ENDOMETRIOSIS

Endometriosis is a common, often chronic condition in which glandular tissue that is normally found only in the uterine lining is found outside the uterus. Common locations for this glandular tissue are along the back of the cervix and around the Fallopian tubes and ovaries. The glands "cycle" with the menstrual cycle and can cause monthly internal bleeding, typically causing severe pain with menses that gets worse as scar tissue forms where bleeding has occurred. Other common problems are pain during sexual intercourse, infertility, or ovarian cysts.

Endometriosis has been called "the career woman's disease" since it seems to be more common in women who have not been pregnant. But it can occur in any woman.

The diagnosis can be very difficult to make since many women with pain do *not* have endometriosis and many women with endometriosis have no symptoms. For women who have chronic pain, a doctor may suggest a laparoscopy, a surgical procedure in which a viewing instrument is placed in the abdomen to help make a diagnosis.

The treatments available for endometriosis are not wonderful. Surgery may be required to remove large chunks of glandular tissue or scar tissue. The only "cure" is a hysterectomy. A male hormone, danazol, will help temporarily but may cause side effects (weight gain, acne, facial hair). Birth control pills may help but cannot be used indefinitely in women over 35 or in smokers. Progestins can help.

Recently, a hormone (Luteinizing Hormone Releasing Hormone, or LHRH) that creates an artificial menopause has been tried with some success, but it is unclear if this is safe or effective for long-term use.

Surgery can be helpful. For mild cases, sometimes cautery, or laser or surgical removal of the tissue may help. For severe cases, hysterectomy and removal of the ovaries may be the only solution.

Women who have or suspect they have endometriosis may want to contact local women's centers to learn about support groups.

Happily, menopause often brings an end to endometriosis symptoms!

PELVIC INFLAMMATORY DISEASE (PID)

Pelvic inflamatory disease refers to a common condition in which the uterus, Fallopian tubes, and in some cases the ovaries and surrounding lower abdominal structures become inflamed. PID can be caused by a variety of organisms, including gonorrhea, chlamydia, or bacteria normally found in the intestine. Frequently, several different organisms are responsible. (Read more in chapter 10 about sexually transmitted diseases and how they can lead to PID.)

PID is practically nonexistent in women who are not sexually active. It is much more common in women who have multiple partners (or whose *partners* have multiple partners!). Intrauterine devices (IUDs) increase both susceptibility to PID and the severity of the infections.

Typical symptoms may range from mild lower abdominal aching to pain with intercourse to severe pain and high temperatures. PID can be very difficult to diagnose, since the symptoms can be similar to those of endometriosis, appendicitis, or bowel problems, such as diverticulitis or irritable bowel syndrome.

PID can block the Fallopian tubes and cause infertility; it can cause serious illness and even death.

If you think you might have PID, seek medical attention. A doctor may do cervical cultures (though these are only of limited use since bacteria may be causing problems internally and not culture out of the cervix). If the case seems mild, the doctor may suggest oral antibiotics. If the diagnosis is in doubt or the infection seems serious, you may need hospitalization to have intravenous antibiotics and observation. If you have had recurrent episodes of PID, sometimes hysterectomy and removal of infected tubes, and even ovaries, may be the only way to get rid of the pain.

DILATATION AND CURETTAGE (D AND C)

A D and C is a minor surgical procedure sometimes recommended for women who have heavy menses or bleeding after menopause. The cervix is dilated and the wall of the uterus is scraped (curetted). This can be an excellent diagnostic/therapeutic procedure for evaluating abnormal bleeding and removing tissue growth in the uterine lining.

At times, an office procedure called an endometrial biopsy or aspiration may be substituted for the D and C, which may require hospitalization and anesthesia.

HYSTERECTOMY

In the Holt-Kahn survey group, 29.7% of the women had had hysterectomies. Many others commented that they are considering hysterectomy. Some requested information that would allow them to talk more knowledgeably about this subject with their doctors. Some complained about being pressured by their doctors.

"Include enough information so that women can feel they will be able to talk to doctors as equals with facts at their fingertips when it becomes necessary to

discuss the possibility of a hysterectomy. The male gynecologists I've seen over the years act like gods and expect the women to agree to everything without question. I questioned my current one a lot and he finally realized he had to discuss things, not just make pronouncements!"

"I'd like to see the latest research on hysterectomies. My doctor plans to do one on me as a preventative of cervical cancer."

In this section you will find definitions of some terms you should know (more in the Glossary), questions you should ask, and specific indications (and nonindications) for surgery.

Terms You Should Know:

HYSTERECTOMY. Removal of the uterus. "Total" hysterectomy technically refers to removal of all of the uterus, including the cervix, while "partial" hysterectomy refers to removal of only part of the uterus. "Partial" hysterectomies are rarely done, since there is little advantage in leaving the cervix behind, although occasionally scar tissue or heavy bleeding may necessitate leaving the cervix.

But it is not this simple. Lay terminology often confuses "total" and "partial," using "total" to refer to removal of the uterus, Fallopian tubes, and ovaries. In medical terms, this is called a "total hysterectomy, bilateral salpingo-oophorectomy." Laypersons often refer to removal of the uterus alone as a "partial" hysterectomy, a confusion that may be subtly encouraged by doctors trying to make the surgery seem more palatable. *Be specific with your doctor about which organs he or she means when talking about surgery.*

OOPHORECTOMY. Removal of an ovary. "Bilateral" means both ovaries, "salpingo-oophorectomy" means Fallopian tubes and ovaries, which are often removed together because they are closely attached.

FIBROID OR LEIOMYOMA. A common fibrous growth in the muscle wall of the uterus; 30 to 50% of all women develop fibroids. Fibroids most commonly occur in the 40 to 50 age group. Fibroids can cause bleeding or pain, but most often cause no symptoms.

MYOMECTOMY. Removal of fibroids. A myomectomy can be an alternative to a hysterectomy. However, because fibroids can recur and the myomectomy can be as major a form of surgery as a hysterectomy, a myomectomy is not commonly performed unless a woman wants more children.

VAGINAL HYSTERECTOMY. Removal of the uterus through the vagina.

ABDOMINAL HYSTERECTOMY. Removal of the uterus through an abdominal incision, usually either up-and-down from the navel to the pubic bone or crosswise an inch or so above the pubic bone.

INCIDENTAL APPENDECTOMY. Removal of the appendix at the time of gynecologic surgery. A few gynecologists do this; you certainly should know if yours plans to do so.

QUESTIONS TO ASK BEFORE HAVING A HYSTERECTOMY

Why Are You Having a Hysterectomy?

As one woman commented, "If you are wondering why you need the surgery, you probably don't!" With the exception of early, asymptomatic cervical or uterine cancers detected on screening exams, most indications for hysterectomy cause symptoms.

Heavy vaginal bleeding that causes anemia and does not respond to hormonal therapy or a simpler D and C (scraping of the uterine wall) is a good reason for surgery.

Enormous, rapidly growing fibroids that cause pressure and increasing abdominal girth, or severely painful endometriosis that does not respond to other forms of therapy, may also be good reasons for surgery. Women who have pain or bleeding rarely doubt the need for surgery; in fact, they are usually banging at the gynecologist's door demanding it. It is the women who feel fine but are told they have small fibroids or "relaxation" of the pelvic organs who may doubt the need for surgery—as well they should!

Several studies have shown that hysterectomy rates seem to reflect the supply and payment mechanisms for surgeons rather than medical need (John Bunker, "Surgical Manpower," *New England Journal of Medicine* 282 [1970]: p. 3; Rita Nickerson et al., "Doctors Who Perform Operations," *New England Journal of Medicine* 295 [1976]: pp. 921–926; John Bunker, "Elective Hysterectomy, Pro and Con," *New England Journal of Medicine* 295 [1976]: pp. 264–268). Rates of hysterectomy are higher when doctors make money from doing surgery (fee-for-service medicine). Hysterectomy rates vary widely from country to country and within regions of the United States, without any evidence that women in high-rate areas are sicker or that women in low-rate areas are dying of untreated diseases.

If the reason for surgery is not immediately obvious to you, you would do well to question the surgeon.

What Are the Alternatives to Hysterectomy?

Often a good alternative to hysterectomy is to do nothing.

Small, asymptomatic fibroids can simply be rechecked at frequent intervals. Women who have heavy periods should be checked for anemia with a blood test, and possibly for early uterine cancer with a Pap smear and sampling of the uterine lining, but can often take vitamin and iron supplements and eat well to counteract the draining effects of the blood loss. Situations causing abnormal Pap smears can sometimes be treated with lesser procedures.

Your doctor may have good reasons for not recommending these alternatives in your case, but he or she should certainly be willing to discuss alternatives and give good reasons why they may not be appropriate for you.

Should You Get a Second Opinion?

If you have any reason to question your doctor's recommendation, or if you do not know the doctor well, the answer is probably yes. Many insurance companies *require* second opinions prior to elective surgery and maintain lists of well-trained, independent specialists who have a track record of sound judgments. Diane Scully, in *Men Who Control Women's Health* (Boston: Houghton Mifflin, 1980), cites an unpublished report by Eugene McCarthy to the AMA Commission on the Cost of Medical Care that showed that 43% of recommendations for elective hysterectomy were not confirmed by a second opinion. In the case of diagnosed neoplastic disease, the second opinion should be from a gynecologic oncologist.

There are two important limitations to second opinions. The first is that since gynecologic training is surgically oriented, gynecologists are trained to perform hysterectomies for a wide variety of indications that may or may not be "necessary." You might have to see many different doctors before you find a qualified physician who is open-minded about alternatives to surgery. Sometimes a nonsurgical physician such as an internist or family practitioner may be a good source of a second opinion, although he or she may not recognize the seriousness of an abnormality, or, conversely, may be less willing to "wait and see" what direction an abnormality may take.

The second limitation is that there are legitimate differences of opinion among conscientious, well-trained doctors. The fact that a second opinion does not confirm the first doctor's recommendation does not mean the first doctor is a quack! It may mean that the second doctor is overly conservative about surgery, or that your case is in a gray area—which is a good reason for seeking third and fourth opinions! Even though doctors tend to be suspicious of patients who do a lot of "doctor shopping," the advantage to you is that you will probably find a doctor with whom you feel very comfortable.

Should Your Ovaries Be Removed?

> *"It was tough because my ovaries were removed without any discussion before surgery, and so it was instant menopause."*

In the Holt-Kahn survey group, nearly half the hysterectomized women also had their ovaries removed. Traditional gynecologic practice has been to remove ovaries at the time of hysterectomy on women over age 40. The theory behind this is that the ovaries do not have very long to function anyway, and that removal eliminates the risk of ovarian cancer—a disease that will affect approximately one out of a hundred women and that is usually widespread when detected and usually fatal.

In the Holt-Kahn survey, 26.5% of the women gynecologists have had their ovaries removed, in contrast to 13.4% of the total sample. This may reflect a cancer phobia on the part of the people who must treat women with ovarian cancer. Other reasons for removing the ovaries are primary ovarian disease such as endometriosis or recurrent cyst formation.

There are also valid reasons for leaving the ovaries in place, both because they continue to be active hormonally in some women well into their fifties and certainly are a more natural source of hormones than pills or creams, and because many women object philosophically to having normal female reproductive organs removed. The pros and cons are summarized in the accompanying box.

Enlarged ovaries

A hormonal imbalance can cause a normal follicle or corpus luteum to enlarge and form a cyst. Cysts in the ovaries are not uncommon during the reproductive years.

One type of ovarian cyst, a dermoid, is rather interesting. Usually benign, these may contain hair, fat, even teeth! Needless to say, dermoids (medically called "mature teratomas") require surgery lest they rupture into the abdomen or become "torsed" (twisted) and destroy the ovary.

Your physician may use ultrasonography to aid in the diagnosis of an ovarian cyst. Sometimes oral contraceptives are prescribed to shrink cysts. Large cysts may or may not cause pain. Chronic pelvic pain may result from a variety of causes, and before surgery is performed other causes should be ruled out.

Prior to menopause, most cysts are fluid-filled and will disappear on their own. However, if an ovarian mass does *not* disappear, or if a woman is past or in menopause, it may have to be removed surgically. Although most ovarian masses are benign in young women, a significant proportion of enlarged ovaries in older women will be cancerous. Hence, in older women, doctors usually insist on removing enlarged ovaries.

Reasons for Leaving Ovaries in at the Time of Hysterectomy:

- No artificial, premature menopause
- No need for replacement hormones (at least until a woman might consider them, the time of natural menopause)
- Philosophical preference for not removing normal tissue
- Removal would make surgery riskier (may be the case with vaginal hysterectomy or if ovaries are normal but surrounded by scar tissue)

Reasons for Removing Ovaries:

- Ovarian disease (severe endometriosis or pelvic inflammatory disease, recurrent cysts, or precancerous or cancerous conditions)
- Strong family history of ovarian cancer or disabling fear of developing ovarian cancer
- Ovaries have ceased functioning or will probably wind down in the near future (Obviously, this is a subjective matter and an educated guess at what constitutes the near future.)

In summary, regarding removal of ovaries, there is no simple answer. One woman at age 39 might choose to have her ovaries removed if she has had recurrent problems with endometriosis or ovarian cysts. Another woman might choose to have her ovaries left in at age 49 if they are normal and she is philosophically opposed to removal of normal tissue and willing to accept the risk of ovarian cancer. Recognize that this is an issue some doctors feel strongly about, and, if you and your doctor are at loggerheads over the issue, it is important that you find a reputable doctor who is willing to honor your feelings.

Should You Have a Vaginal or an Abdominal Hysterectomy?

A vaginal hysterectomy has many advantages: Typically, recovery is faster, there is less pain, and many women find the lack of an abdominal scar makes the psychological adaptation to surgery easier. Unfortunately, several conditions contraindicate vaginal hysterectomy. These include large uterine fibroids; suspected ovarian disease; suspected scar tissue due to previous surgery, endometriosis, or pelvic inflammatory disease; or a tight vaginal opening. Generally, these exclusions leave only women who have borne children vaginally, have smallish uteri, and otherwise normal pelvic organs. In this group, vaginal hysterectomies are recommended for women whose Pap smears are abnormal or who have uterine prolapse or intractable bleeding from a small or minimally enlarged uterus. Most of the women requiring hysterectomies have large fibroids or a lot of scar tissue and hence must have an abdominal procedure. Generally, there just aren't that many women with small uteri and normal pelvic anatomy who really must have hysterectomies!

If you are in doubt, or your doctor's reason does not sound logical, get more opinions! Surgeons vary greatly in their philosophy toward and skills at vaginal surgery; some surgeons with a great deal of experience may feel comfortable with a tricky vaginal hysterectomy, while other surgeons might not.

Can You Pre-Bank Your Own Blood or Have a Family Member Donate Blood for Use During Your Surgery?

Most hysterectomy patients do not require blood transfusions, but between 1% and 10% do, and if you are anemic prior to surgery or have large fibroids or much scar tissue, your chances of needing blood may be much greater. Due to concern about hepatitis and AIDS from blood transfusions, many women are requesting to donate some of their own blood in advance in case it is needed at surgery. Unfortunately, women who are having surgery because of heavy bleeding may not be able to get their blood counts up high enough to safely self-donate, and not all blood banks are equipped to handle self-directed donations.

Directed donations from friends and family members are trickier, since the blood must not cross-react with your own, and some blood banks fear that family members under duress to donate blood may actually be riskier donors than healthy, altruistic volunteers.

Fortunately, current screening tests for hepatitis and AIDS make volunteer donor blood reasonably safe. You certainly should discuss with your doctor, however, the odds for needing a transfusion in your particular case and the availability of self- and directed-donor programs in your area.

What Are the Potential Complications of Surgery?

Hysterectomy is not a benign procedure! A study from Cornell University estimated that 1,700 deaths resulted from 787,000 hysterectomies performed in 1975 (.2%). That study estimated that 22% of these hysterectomies may have been unnecessary. (Diane Scully, *Men Who Control Women's Health* [Boston: Houghton Mifflin, 1980]). Injury to the ureters (tubes from the kidney to the bladder) that usually requires further surgery and can involve lifelong urinary problems occur in 0.5% to 2.5% of hysterectomies, according to the American College of Obstetricians and Gynecologists (*ACOG Technical Bulletin* 83 [January 1985]). Injuries to the bowel can occur on occasion, requiring a colostomy or further reparative surgery. Some 30 to 50% of women may suffer "morbidity" from surgery, most often in the form of postoperative fevers requiring antibiotic treatment.

Your doctor should be honest about these potential complications and willing to give you realistic odds in your particular situation. Fortunately, major complications are relatively rare. Unfortunately, the more indicated the surgery (severe scar tissue, huge fibroids) the higher the complication rate will be. Surgeons have a difficult job in warning about potential complications, since courts have held doctors liable for both failing to warn about potential complications and for scaring people so much that they failed to have needed surgery done!

How Many of These Operations Has Your Doctor Performed, and What Is His or Her Personal Complication Rate?

This is a hard question to ask, and a threatening one for doctors to answer, but an honest, conscientious doctor should be able to give you a straight answer.

There is no "right" answer to this question; you basically want to know that your doctor feels comfortable with the recommended surgery and does not seem evasive. Realize that a young, new doctor may be highly competent but not very experienced. Realize that a surgeon with widely known skills may get more difficult cases and have a higher complication rate, and that a surgeon could have a low complication rate because he or she does a lot of very simple (and possibly unnecessary) cases. Realize that if your surgeon works at a teaching hospital a relatively inexperienced resident may be participating in your surgery—a price you pay for the extra staffing, up-to-date methods, and quality controls often found at teaching hospitals. Realize that a less competent physician may underestimate his or her complication rate, while a competent physician is likelier to be honest with you. Given these limitations, the answer to this question must be put into perspective, but the answer will at least give you some insight into your risks.

What Is Your Doctor's Reputation in the Community?

This is obviously not a question for your doctor, but for your friends and medical acquaintances. Certainly there are wonderful, competent doctors who may be a little out of the mainstream. Certainly there are marginally competent physicians who may be prominent due to their personalities or social activities. But, in general, doctors with good reputations among their patients and colleagues have come by those reputations by taking good care of their patients.

BREAST PROBLEMS

In the Holt-Kahn survey group, 18% of women reported having had breast surgery. More than 62% have had mammograms.

The most common complaints about breasts are size, pain, discharge, and lumps.

Size only becomes a medical problem if a woman is contemplating surgery for augmentation or reduction or if heavy breasts cause back problems. Any woman contemplating cosmetic surgery should be sure that her reasons are valid and her goals and expectations realistic, and that she can afford the surgery and has a competent plastic surgeon. Goals such as looking better in clothes or alleviating back pain from heavy breasts are realistic.

Breast surgery leaves scars. Breast implants feel a bit different than normal breast tissue. Women should look at a surgeon's "before" and "after" pictures as well as those in plastic surgery textbooks, recognizing that a surgeon will photograph and exhibit his best, not his worst, work. Realize that few insurance policies will cover elective breast surgery, although most policies will cover reconstructive surgery after a mastectomy, and breast reduction to correct a back problem.

As for checking the credentials of your plastic surgeon, find out where he or she was educated, if he or she is certified by the Board of the American College of Plastic and Reconstructive Surgery and/or American College of Surgeons. If at all possible, talk to other women who have had similar surgery about the competency of their surgeon, if there were complications, and if they were satisfied with the results. Also, seek referrals from various cancer organizations and women's resource centers.

Breast Cancer

Most women are terrified of breast cancer. There is probably not a midlife woman in America who has not had a close friend or relative with this dreaded disease. Breast cancer is frighteningly common, can attack any woman, and is disfiguring and frequently fatal. Small wonder that women are terrified of any lump, bump, or pain in their breasts. But there is finally some good news: New ways of diagnosing and treating breast cancer offer improved cure rates and less disfiguring treatments. Preventive diets may reduce the rate of disease.

The good news about breast diseases: Most breast lumps and bumps and pains are not due to cancer. There are several common and benign conditions that account for lumps and pains.

Fibrocystic Disease

"Fibrocystic disease" is a disorder in which the breasts are lumpy and painful, often in cyclic fashion, with the worst pain just prior to menstruation. It is arguable whether fibrocystic breasts truly are a disease or simply a normal, if uncomfortable, variant. A few women have disabling pain, but for most women, fibrocystic breasts are a nuisance and occasional source of alarm since prominent lumps can occur. Women who have fibrocystic breasts may have to rely on mammography and periodic removal of cysts by aspiration (fluid withdrawal) or biopsy, since it is impossible to guarantee that any persistent lump is not cancerous.

Several measures may improve fibrocystic breasts, including using oral contraceptives, avoiding caffeine and similar substances (often found in cold capsules, asthma medication, and diet pills), and taking Vitamin E supplements. For severe cases, a male-type hormone, danazol, may be effective, although side effects may occur. And, finally, fibrocystic disease often improves with menopause and the cessation of the menstrual cycle, although some women find that the condition temporarily gets worse during the hormonal changes of their early forties. The condition should be considered more serious in women whose mother, grandmother, or sisters have had breast cancer.

Breast Discharge

Breast discharge should be called to the attention of your doctor! Causes of breast discharge include frequent nipple stimulation, pituitary disorders, benign growths, and cancers. The vast majority of breast discharges are not due to cancer, but this symptom should be evaluated. Your doctor may recommend pituitary testing, sending a sample of the discharge to the lab, or a mammogram or biopsy.

Breast Pain

Breast pain not related to obvious fibrocystic disease is a common complaint, and its cause is often unclear. Certainly a woman with pain should have a careful exam and possibly a mammogram. Most such breast pain, which women may describe as a "hot" or "burning" sensation, may be caused by glandular activity or inflammation of normal breast tissue. Breast infections and abscesses can occur, but are not very common in women who are not breast-feeding. Sometimes muscle strain from exercising or lifting can cause breast pain. A blow to the chest or poorly fitting bra can also be the culprit. Unless there is an infection or benign or malignant growth, most breast pain may have no obvious treatment other than following the suggestions for fibrocystic breasts and using mild painkillers.

Breast Enlargement

Breast enlargement is a common complaint of women in their forties. This can be due to simple weight gain or to continuous estrogen stimulation. Some women have breast enlargement when they start taking replacement hormones; this is usually dose-related and will improve if the estrogen dose is gradually lowered. Equally common is the complaint of breast "shrinkage" or "sagging." This is due to a combination of loss of hormones, poor muscle tone, and the wear and the tear of aging. Upper arm exercises and a good support bra will help. Some women find that estrogen replacement therapy seems to make their breasts feel fuller, and a few women resort to plastic surgery to correct this problem. The best solution is probably to recognize that it is your positive feelings about yourself, not minor variations in the tilt of your breasts, that is most important.

Breast Self-Examination and Mammography

During regular gynecological examinations, most doctors ask: "Do you examine your breasts regularly yourself?" Your answer should be yes. If you would like additional information on the technique recommended by the American College of Obstetricians and Gynecologists, you may write to:

ACOG
600 Maryland Avenue, SW, Suite 300 East
Washington, DC 20024-2588

You may also obtain information from:

American Cancer Society
90 Park Avenue
New York, New York 10016

Mammography

Mammography is gaining increasing acceptance as an adjunct diagnostic procedure. It is used in addition to self-exam and examination by a physician to detect early changes in breast tissue.

A major multicenter study by the American Cancer Society-National Cancer Institute Breast Cancer Detection Demonstration Projects indicates that "one-third of the breast cancers occurred in women between the ages of 35 and 49 years, and most of these lesions were either in situ or did not involve the regional lymph nodes. Most of the cancers were detected by mammography, and a much higher percentage were detected by mammography alone than by physical examination alone" (*CA—A Cancer Journal for Clinicians* 33 [July-August 1983]).

The American Cancer Society recommends the following for asymptomatic women: (1) Baseline mammogram, ages 35 to 40. (2) "That the Cancer-Related Checkup Guidelines for breast cancer detection be modified for asymptomatic women age 40 to 49 years. Women in this age group should have a physical examination of the breast annually, and mammography should be performed at intervals of one to two years." (3) Yearly mammograms after age 50.

At current radiation levels, risks are minimal. Be sure your local mammography facility uses up-to-date equipment with minimal radiation exposure (one rad or less per breast).

And don't overdepend on mammography. Continue self-exams and medical checkups. Even with a normal mammogram, suspicious lumps should be biopsied. A combination of self-exam, regular examination by your doctor, and regular mammography will pick up tumors at the earliest and most treatable stage.

Mammography is only about 85 to 90% accurate. One study estimated it as low as 69%. It is *essential* that women become alert to this and *do not allow* a physician to "watch" a lump without biopsy. This is particularly important for younger women and those who are pregnant. Such women should seek out a competent breast specialist or a well-qualified surgeon and not rely on the mammogram alone. Also, the value of mammography depends on the radiologist reading and interpreting it, as well as the technician who takes the picture.

When you find a lump

The normal breast feels glandular, and many women use this as an excuse for relying on their doctor, the mammogram, or Lady Luck to find lumps. The reason for doing self-examination is to get used to your own glandular pattern so when you feel that pebbly, rocklike feeling of a cancer you will recognize it as being different from your normal breast tissue. (However, there are several kinds of nodules that feel different. A benign lump can also appear rocklike. Doctors who examine you every few months may not pick up cancers as early as you can!)

After finding a lump, most women go to see their family doctor or gynecologist. The doctor will examine the breast, ask about the time of your menstrual cycle, pain or other symptoms, and possibly order a mammogram. If the lump feels like a cyst, the doctor may suggest waiting a week or two or until after your next period to recheck it, or may suggest "aspirating" (drawing the fluid out of) the cyst. The fluid may be checked for malignant cells. A woman may be referred to a general surgeon or breast specialist for this procedure, although many family doctors and OB/GYNs may aspirate cysts in the office. If the lump is suspicious, the mammogram is suspicious, the lump does not disappear after aspiration, or the aspirated fluid looks bloody or creamy (normal cysts have clear, slightly yellow-tinged fluid), the doctor will probably recommend a biopsy of the lump. In the United States, gynecologists generally do not do breast surgery; they usually refer patients to a general surgeon.

If no fluid is found or if the lump does not feel cystic, it should be biopsied. This is often done with a local anesthestic in the doctor's office or as outpatient surgery in a hospital. Several states have laws requiring that women must be counseled about alternatives to mastectomy for breast cancer. Also, having the biopsy performed separately means that the tissue interpretation can be done in leisurely, painstaking fashion. At times, with the old "one-step" procedure, the final biopsy reading did not even show cancer!

Keep in mind that there are still many surgeons who insist on a "one-step" procedure. The patient must question the doctor about procedure. There are doctors who still almost always perform modified radical mastectomies and will not seriously consider any alternative.

Warnings

Do *not* ignore lumps, even if your mammogram is negative. Get to know your own breasts. Women who self-examine often detect masses that doctors miss.

Don't hide your head in the sand! Many women are "afraid" to check their breasts, but cancers found late will generally require radical surgery and chemotherapy. If the cancer has spread by the time you find it, your chance of surviving five years is 45%; if the cancer is confined to the breast, the five-year survival chance is 85% (Douglas Marchant, "Epidemiology of Breast Cancer," *Clinical Obstetrics and Gynecology* 25 [1982]: pp. 387). The *cure* rate for breast cancer found late is low: 80% of breast cancer patients not dying of other causes will die of their disease within 25 years. Most health care professionals expect that increasing rates of self-exam, mammograms, and biopsies will result in earlier detection and improved survival over the next 20 years.

Once a cancer is found: Then what?

Talk to people. Isolation is your worst enemy. Talk to any medical professionals you know and to any friends who have had personal experiences. Reach out and talk to:

Gynecologists
Family doctor
Nurses
Friends who have had breast cancers or close contact with a patient

Volunteer groups, such as Y-ME and Reach to Recovery
Local hospitals or local branches of American Cancer Society
   may be contacted for names of recovery groups
National Cancer Institute
State Cancer Councils

Why all this talking? Because within two to three weeks, you will need to become educated about many different areas—breast cancer treatment is in a state of flux and is confusing and controversial. Issues that you will need to learn about are:

YOUR AGE If you are premenopausal, you may be more likely to receive chemotherapy, and breast cancers in young women are often more aggressive (fast-growing).

STAGING If your cancer is very, very early, the tumor is small—less than one centimeter (smaller than your little fingernail), and your lymph nodes are negative for malignancy, you might be a candidate for less disfiguring procedures.

CELL TYPES Certain cell types can be more aggressive or are likelier to occur in both breasts, which might influence your doctor toward recommending chemotherapy and/or doing a biopsy on the other breast.

RECEPTOR STATUS Your cancer should be tested for estrogen and progesterone receptors, because if these exist and you need chemotherapy, antiestrogens may be used that have only minor side effects (vaginal dryness, hot flashes) rather than the nausea, hair loss, and illness often associated with other chemotherapy.

LYMPH NODES Probably one of the most important prognostic (predictive) factors about breast cancer is whether or not cancer cells are found in the lymph nodes. In general, if the nodes are all negative, the chances for cure are good (85% five-year survival); the National Surgical Adjuvant Breast Project found only a 13% ten-year survival rate if more than four nodes tested out positive. Premenopausal women with positive nodes unquestionably benefit from chemotherapy. The results in postmenopausal women are not as obvious, although if nodes are positive and receptor studies are positive, the response rate (decrease in recurrences) is good with use of anti-estrogens (National Institutes of Health Consensus Conference, *Journal of the American Medical Society* 254 [1985]: pp. 3461).

Breast cancer treatment

Because there are so many technical and complicated issues in breast cancer treatment, you need to talk to many people to get an overview of what your options may be and, even more important, to identify a surgeon and medical facility that are first and foremost competent to care for you and sensitive and up-to-date concerning options.

Much of the confusion and controversy about breast cancer treatment has come in the form of criticism of the surgical treatment. The "traditional" surgeries include:

- *Radical mastectomy (Halsted procedure)* Removal of breast, both pectoralis muscles, axillary lymph nodes; used now for large tumors and tumors attached to the chest wall. The Halsted procedure is a kind of "gold standard" against which other treatments are measured. The Urban procedure or "extended radical" includes removal of lymph nodes under the mediastinum (inner chest wall) and is rarely done.
- *"Modified radical"* Removal of breast, pectoralis minor, and lymph nodes. This is the most frequently used procedure.
- *Simple mastectomy* (with or without lymph nodes) Removal of breast used for *very* early cancers or precancers, or for severe breast disease.

Recently, there has been much interest among women in lesser procedures, specifically:

- *Quadrantectomy* Removal of about one-quarter of the breast (the "quadrant" in which a cancer is located).
- *Lumpectomy* Lumpectomy or wide excisional biopsy may be an option for very early cancers, but surgeons must be able to feel the cancer easily or be guided by a needle or dye placed in a mammographic lesion. In general, studies to date have shown that for very early cancers, lumpectomy and lymph node sampling plus radiation has comparable five-year survival rates to modified radical mastectomy. But figures on longer survival are not available and many breast surgeons are firmly convinced that a modified radical mastectomy remains the best treatment.

Women eager to have effective, nondisfiguring treatments for breast cancer have been sharply critical of the lack of such options. There are some good (and some bad) reasons why progress seems so slow:

- Breast cancer carries such a high mortality rate that doctors are reluctant to experiment and possibly risk women's lives.

- The split between surgeons responsible for surgery, radiation therapists responsible for radiation, and medical oncologists responsible for chemotherapy, has, in many cases, limited interdisciplinary experimentation to large high-volume centers.
- The long time frame of the disease means that the risks and benefits of a new treatment may not be clear until 20 years after it comes into widescale use.

The vast majority of doctors involved in breast cancer treatment are men. They may have trouble relating to the issues of body image and sexuality in a 55-year-old woman. Many women do not feel doctors give sufficient weight to the issue of body image.

Surgeons are basically a conservative group. They are reluctant to depart from the beaten track and open themselves to criticism and lawsuits over poor results from less standard procedures.

Realize also that radiation is no piece of cake. Adjuvant radiation involves several weeks of frequent hospital visits, and while it is initially less disfiguring than mastectomy, some women will develop stiffened skin months or years later.

Adjuvant chemotherapy for postmenopausal women is controversial. According to a National Institutes of Health (NIH) Consensus Conference report published in the *Journal of the American Medical Association* (December 26, 1985), while adjuvant chemotherapy has demonstrated a significant increase in disease-free survival as well as a significant reduction in death in *pre*menopausal women with breast cancer, the usefulness of adjuvant chemotherapy for *post*menopausal women is less well established.

The new NIH recommendations are: For premenopausal women with evidence of cancer spread to lymph nodes, regardless of hormone receptor status, treatment with established combination chemotherapy should become standard care; for premenopausal patients without lymph node involvement, adjuvant chemotherapy is not generally recommended (it should be considered only for certain high-risk patients in this group).

For postmenopausal women with positive nodes and positive hormone-receptor levels, the anti-estrogen hormone compound tamoxifen is the treatment of choice; for postmenopausal women with positive nodes and negative hormone-receptor levels, chemotherapy cannot be recommended as standard practice, although it may be considered; for postmenopausal women with no evidence of lymph node involvement, regardless of hormone receptor levels, there is no indication for routine adjuvant treatment.

Further studies are under way and many issues require additional investigation. Each case should be individually evaluated and treatment planned accordingly.

Because of all these factors, even though a woman would like a flexible surgeon willing to perform and experienced in lumpectomies, she may have trouble finding one. Many surgeons feel strongly that modified radical remains the "gold standard" and will do lumpectomies only under protest and with misgivings. Understandably, many women are in a state of shock and likely to numbly follow their doctor's advice. Therefore, we may continue to see modified radicals as the standard treatment for some time. Only after many years, after longer follow-up is available on women who had lumpectomies and after more and more tumors are "occult" (found on mammogram only), can we expect to see a trend toward minimal surgery.

The "take home" messages of this section are: Have mammograms! Self-examine! Eat a low-fat diet! (High dietary fat intake seems to play a promoting role in breast cancer development.)

Breast reconstruction after mastectomy

"Breast reconstruction can help a woman look more attractive and make her feel more comfortable in activities where an external prosthesis may be awkward. Additionally, reconstruction can help her reestablish her self-image and self-esteem," says Ann Marcou, co-founder of the Y-ME Breast Cancer Support Program, Homewood, Illinois, which was founded in 1978. Ms. Marcou, a midlife woman and breast cancer patient, has a master's degree in therapeutic counseling from Governors State University, University Park, Illinois. "Breast reconstruction does not cause recurrence of breast cancer and does not interfere with the detection of such recurrence if it happens," says Marcou.

There are a variety of surgical procedures performed in the field of breast reconstruction. Postmastectomy breast reconstruction is one of the most common procedures in the practice of many plastic surgeons, even though the most frequently used techniques are less than two decades old.

"Virtually anyone who desires it can have reconstruction regardless of the type of mastectomy," says Robert M. Swartz, M.D., F.A.C.S., a plastic and reconstructive surgeon in Arlington Heights, Illinois, who goes on to say: "However, it is generally not advisable to perform reconstruction on women who have advanced breast disease, or those with local recurrence at the original surgical site."

In some cases, factors such as extensive skin changes from radiotherapy, extreme thinning of the skin, and loss of the pectoralis muscle make reconstruction more difficult. However, newer procedures enable reconstruction for many women who previously would not have been good candidates.

"Reconstructive surgical procedures generally do not compromise necessary treatment. Detection of recurrence after a properly performed reconstruction is not more difficult following reconstruction, nor is the treatment of such recurrence impaired," comments Dr. Swartz.

For some women, reconstruction can be done at the time of mastectomy, although many surgeons prefer later reconstruction on technical grounds. "More often it is best to wait a few months before the reconstruction procedure. We believe that better reconstructions can be performed after time is allowed for the softening and healing of the mastectomy site. After healing of the area, proper and more predictable placement of breast implants can be obtained," says Dr. Swartz.

The theory has also been advanced that women will adapt better psychologically if they first "mourn" the missing breast and then adapt to the reconstruction. However, most studies have indicated that women probably fare better psychologically with immediate reconstruction.

There's also the problem that most women who have had mastectomies so detest the thought of more surgery that they decide against later reconstruction—even though they would *like* reconstruction, they don't want to go through two or three more operations. Meanwhile, the women who had immediate reconstruction get on with their lives and have the surgery *behind* them. If a woman is seeking the best possible cosmetic results and doesn't mind several surgeries over several months, delayed reconstruction is a good choice. For the woman who wants to get the surgery over quickly and get on with her life, immediate reconstruction (when possible) is a good choice. "My reconstruction was done five years after bilateral mastectomy. It was done entirely in one procedure, including nipple and areola," says Marcou.

Rebuilding the breast consists of reconstructing the absent mound, nipple, and areola. It may include surgery on the remaining breast for its preventive removal or reshaping. This often can be accomplished in one stage, but in some cases may require several operative stages for completion, depending on each patient's physical condition.

"The extent of the original mastectomy somewhat determines the complexity and number of operative stages required for reconstruction," says Dr. Swartz. "Generally, more satisfactory reconstructions can be done for women who have had a modified radical mastectomy, in which the pectoral (chest) muscle is saved but the axillary lymph nodes in the armpit are removed."

"Saving the pectoralis major muscle is important," emphasizes Dr. Swartz. This is the large, fan-shaped muscle that lies beneath the breast and also makes up the fullness of the upper chest and the front of the underarm. "Its presence allows for a more natural appearing reconstruction."

TYPES OF RECONSTRUCTION "The simplest procedures should be done in the fewest number of stages," says Dr. Swartz. There are several general categories of reconstructive procedures:

- Unilateral (one breast) reconstruction
- Reconstruction with alteration of the remaining breast (reducing or reshaping it to match the reconstructed side)
- Reconstruction requiring extra tissue at the mastectomy site
- Reconstruction after prophylactic (preventive) mastectomy
- Immediate reconstruction

Following is an outline of each type of reconstruction.

Unilateral (one breast) reconstruction This procedure:

- Follows total mastectomy or modified radical mastectomy
- Consists of placement of a breast implant beneath the remaining skin and muscle of the chest wall
- Implant may be placed through a portion of the existing mastectomy scar, or through a separate incision beneath the reconstructed breast
- Often the nipple and areolar complex can be reconstructed during the same procedure, although some surgeons prefer later placement of these structures

Reconstruction with alteration of the remaining breast:

- Reduction or lifting of the opposite side so that both breasts will look alike, or as nearly so as possible.
- Sometimes can be completed at a single operative session.

Reconstruction requiring extra tissue at the mastectomy site In this operation:

- More extensive reconstructive procedures are necessary after radical mastectomy, when tumor removal has left a tight skin closure, the chest wall muscles were removed or radiation therapy has been done
- Missing skin and muscle tissue is usually replaced with what is known as the "latissimus dorsi muscle-skin flap" technique

- The flap consists of a large segment of tissue taken from the back, including skin and a large, fan-shaped muscle (latissimus dorsi)
- This tissue is then tunneled through the axillary area onto the front of the chest
- The "donor" scar on the back will be several inches long, but can be placed so that it will be hidden by some bathing suits and low-cut dresses
- Usually a breast implant can be placed at this time
- Nipple and areolar reconstruction is often deferred for several months

Another method for adding extra breast tissue This procedure consists of the following:

- For some women who are appropriate candidates, a large amount of skin and fat may be brought up into the chest from the abdomen
- A bonus is a "tummy tuck" operation, in which a section of fat is removed from the abdomen and brought up to the breast. (A disadvantage may be abdominal weakness.)

Immediate postmastectomy reconstruction This operation:

- Depends on certain circumstances, such as tumor type, location, and size
- Demands appropriate teamwork between oncologist, general surgeon, and reconstructive surgeon
- Results may not be as good as in delayed cases; future refinement may be desirable

TYPES OF PROSTHESES Breast prostheses are well tolerated by the body and cause little reaction. Usually, breast reconstructions involve insertion of a prosthesis or "implant" of one of four basic types:

- Silicone gel
- An implant inflated with saline solution
- A biphasic implant, which is a combination of the above two substances
- Polyurethane-covered implants

The choice is usually made by the surgeon, depending on the patient's reconstructive needs.

RECONSTRUCTING THE NIPPLE There are several ways to reconstruct the nipple and areola. Sometimes a portion of the remaining nipple is used. In other cases, the surrounding pigmented skin (areola) is reconstructed from a skin graft taken from elsewhere on the body. The reconstructed nipple-areola complex is usually a satisfactory facsimile, but is rarely identical to the original in size and shape and lacks erectile property.

WHAT TO EXPECT While complications are relatively infrequent, a woman should discuss all possibilities with her reconstructive surgeon before the operation. All surgical procedures carry risks of complications, such as bleeding, infection, poor wound healing, and unsatisfactory scarring.

Ask your reconstructive surgeon how long you will be out of commission after your breast surgery and your reconstructive surgery. Ask what to expect in specific limitations in activity and work after the proposed surgery. Also, ask about follow-up care and whether you should see the reconstructive surgeon, general surgeon, or oncologist.

In the simplest form of mastectomy, the woman may stay in the hospital less than three days. Some operations and revisions are done on an out-patient basis. If the procedure is relatively simple and their occupations are not physically strenuous, some women return to work within a week following reconstruction. After more extensive operations, up to three weeks away from work may be necessary.

Support groups

As with any other crisis, meeting other women who have or have had the same problems makes a woman feel that she is not alone. Many hospitals and women's health centers across the country have programs for breast cancer patients. These include exercise groups, lecture series, and "rap" sessions. If you or a friend has breast cancer and can't find a local group, you may want to obtain information from:

Y-ME Breast Cancer Support Program
1757 Ridge Road
Homewood, Illinois 60430
Phone: (312) 799-8338

Also call the National Cancer Institute's hotline: 1-800-4-CANCER; or the American Cancer Society's hotline: 1-800-ACS-2345.

Call the local unit of the American Cancer Society to obtain information about Reach to Recovery, a nationwide support system for women who have had breast surgery.

URINARY INCONTINENCE

In the Holt-Kahn survey, nearly half of the women admitted to loss of urine (43.8% called it mild; 4.7% severe). This is a little-talked about problem, and one that most women assume is theirs alone.

Why does urinary loss occur? In part, it is due to anatomy. The female combination of a short urethra (tube from the bladder to the urinary opening), upright posture, and loss of normal muscle tone due to childbirth, obesity, age, and general wear and tear combine to make the normal tightening that prevents urinary loss a less efficient process.

In part, it can be due to medications and to bladder stimulants such as caffeine and diet pills. Occasionally it is due to serious diseases such as multiple sclerosis or tumors in the spinal cord.

The most common form of urinary incontinence in women is known as "stress incontinence," since it occurs only under "stress," such as coughing, laughing, or aerobic dancing.

"Urge incontinence" refers to the situation in which, once you feel the urge, you may not even be able to get to the bathroom in time. The common type of stress incontinence is commonly due to weak muscle tone; urge incontinence is often due to medications or an "irritable," overactive bladder. Complete loss of bladder control is an emergency that requires immediate evaluation, as this can result from spinal cord injuries or damage to the nerves that control the bladder.

After you have had a medical evaluation from an internist or family practitioner and tried the self-help measures to no avail, you may want to consult a gynecologist or urologist about therapies. Standard evaluations for incontinence vary widely from place to place, but among the tests a gynecologist or urologic surgeon may recommend are:

- *Urinalysis* This should be standard procedure.
- *Diabetes screening* Frequent urination is a common symptom of diabetes.
- *Thorough physical examination* During the exam, you will be checked for an enlarged uterus that could be pressing on your bladder, and for a cystocoele or urethrocoele, an anatomic bulging of the urethra or bladder into the vagina.
- *Kidney and bladder X rays* An X ray of the kidney, ureters (tubes into the bladder), and bladder, is called an intravenous pyelogram (IVP, for short). Some dye will be injected into your vein. Except for a feeling of heat throughout your body for a few minutes, you won't feel any discomfort during the procedure.
- *Cystoscopy* This is a technique for looking inside the bladder to see if there are any abnormal growths, inflammation, or damage to the

muscle wall of the bladder. A tube is inserted into the urethra, and an evaluation can be made regarding the adequacy of the muscle tone of the urethra.

- *Urodynamic studies* This is a specialized form of cystoscopy during which the resting muscle tone of the bladder and urethra can be measured, and during which the response to a measured amount of fluid can be evaluated. These are useful for distinguishing anatomic incontinence due to loss of muscle tone from bladder irritability, and some physicians swear by them as a route of determining who will benefit from surgery and who from medication. Other physicians believe that a careful medical history, physical examination, and simpler, more widely available tests are sufficient for most cases of incontinence.

Treatments

Nonsurgical treatments (in addition to Kegel exercises [see chapter 2], weight loss, etc.):

- Estrogen therapy may restore some skin tone to an atrophic vaginal area, alleviate urgency due to vaginal atrophy, and help mild stress incontinence.
- Pessaries are vaginal support devices that may return the bladder and urethra to a more normal position and help restore control. (See the section on vaginal relaxation later in this chapter.)
- Women with bladder irritability may improve with use of a class of drugs called anticholinergics (most common example, probanthine) which relax the bladder tone. Sedatives and tranquilizers have been reported as useful for some women, possibly because they don't complain as much to their doctors. While in general we caution against overuse of sedatives and tranquilizers, in this setting they may be useful for a few women. We would hate to see someone who could be helped by them suffer; they might be worth a limited try.
- Surprisingly, a few women may respond to a drug called Urecholine which *increases* bladder tone—these are often women with very weak bladder muscles, such as women who have multiple sclerosis.

Surgical treatments

A variety of surgical treatments are possible, with different ones useful for different individuals. Basically, the procedures are designed to improve muscle tone under the urethra and improve the anatomic location of the bladder and urethra. One approach is to make an abdominal incision above the bladder and tighten the area around the urethra by either sutures or some type of sling. Another technique is to approach the urethra from the vagina and increase the vaginal tone. If the uterus is sliding down into the vagina, or is enlarged or otherwise abnormal, a concurrent hysterectomy may be recommended.

HOW SUCCESSFUL IS SURGERY? "Success" rates vary widely, according to the medical literature. Any one surgical approach will not cure all cases. In published data with properly selected patients, somewhere in the range of 90% of all women will benefit from surgery in the short run. Frequently, however, the problem recurs years later, and the "success" rate after recurrent surgeries is often reduced. Since gynecologists and urologists are trained as surgeons, they may recommend surgery readily, generally citing the published short-term success rates of the best centers. It has been the impression of many women, however, upon informally polling their friends, that actual long-term successes may not be that common. And often doctors who cite high success rates also counsel their patients against activities such as running or aerobics for fear of compromising the surgery—the very reason many women have the surgery is to be able to take part in vigorous activities!

Overall, we would urge surgery only for severe cases. Risks of surgery include death from excess bleeding or anesthesia, and occasionally women have "fistulas," holes in the bladder, as a result of surgery.

Be sure you consider the surgery carefully and select a urologist or gynecologist experienced in these procedures. For most women with only occasional, minor problems, simpler methods are probably as effective.

VAGINAL RELAXATION

Women not infrequently note a sense of vaginal "looseness" or "something sticking out." This is not so much an aging problem per se but rather a problem of stretching during childbirth and general wear and tear on the tissues. Heredity plays a role, since vaginal relaxation is less common in black women and often runs in families. The "something sticking out" of the vagina may be the urethra (urethrocoele), the bladder (cystocoele), the rectum bulging forward (rectocoele), the uterus (uterine prolapse), or frequently some combination of the above. This is not generally dangerous! Occasionally, spotting due to local irritation can result, as can frequent vaginal infections due to tissue irritation, or loss of good bladder or bowel control. Most often, the sensation is mainly an annoyance. Not infrequently, a woman will comment that her husband complains about a loose vagina; often this complaint masks sexual dysfunction rather than an anatomic problem (see chapter 10).

Vaginal relaxation can be aggravated by obesity. In theory, exercises, such as jogging or aerobics, that involve pressure on the pelvic organs would be expected to aggravate relaxation, but, in practice, most women who exercise find that the weight loss and improved overall muscle tone resulting from exercise actually improve their vaginal tone. Women who are concerned about this problem may find that exercises such as swimming or cycling put a little less downward pressure on their pelvic organs. Kegel exercises can help, as can estrogens if atrophy of the vaginal tissues is contributing to the relaxation.

Pessaries

When medical intervention becomes necessary, the choices are either surgical correction or placement of a device called a pessary. Pessaries are vaginal devices usually made of plastic or rubber that hold the uterus and/or vaginal walls in place. They come in a variety of shapes and sizes. One type resembles the rigid edge of a diaphragm and fits behind the cervix and under the pubic bone. One type resembles a bell, with the larger rim placed under the uterus and the smaller dome facing the vagina to facilitate removal. Another type resembles a cube, which allows cervix and vaginal walls to fill in concavities on the surface. Some pessaries may be removed and reinserted by the woman herself; some require inflation and deflation and removal in the doctor's office.

Pessaries can have some minor side effects; some women find themselves more prone to vaginal infections and irritation. Sexual activity is impossible with some types of pessaries in place, so a sexually active woman should discuss this with her doctor in order to choose either a pessary that allows for sexual activity or one that she can remove and replace. Finding a suitable pessary is often a matter of trial and error, and a woman may have to make several trips to the doctor's office due to discomfort, infections, spotting, or the pessary "popping out." Despite these drawbacks, with a little practice, most women with significant prolapse who wish to avoid surgery can eventually find a pessary that helps their prolapse with few or no side effects.

Surgical Repair

Many women prefer a surgical approach to vaginal relaxation. Surgical repair generally consists of removing a wedge of vaginal tissue from the front and back walls of the vagina (anterior and posterior repair) with or without a hysterectomy, depending on the position of the uterus. Immediate surgical results are often quite good, and the vaginal repair itself is fairly minor surgery. However (isn't there always a however?), a hysterectomy is major surgery, and even "minor" vaginal surgery can be complicated by excessive bleeding, damage to the bowel or bladder, and anesthetic complications. In addition to immediate complications, long-term complications can include scar tissue in the vagina or shortening of the vagina that can make intercourse painful, and eventually prolapse of the top of the vagina once the ligaments attached to the uterus are gone. Such complications occur less frequently if an abdominal suspension of the vagina is performed at the time of surgery, but obviously this adds to the surgery itself. Again, it should be obvious that we think surgery should be reserved for only the most severe cases of prolapse and relaxation.

OTHER MAJOR MEDICAL PROBLEMS

Heart disease, diabetes, and arthritis are among many other diseases that affect midlife women. In the Holt-Kahn survey group, 13% reported having high blood pressure, 2.2% had heart disease, and 1.3% had diabetes. Eighteen percent reported that they smoke—a factor implicated in heart disease, lung disease, and diabetes.

Specific information on heart disease, arthritis, diabetes, and the dangers involved in smoking are available from:

American Heart Association
7320 Greenville Avenue
Dallas, Texas 75231

National Heart, Lung, and Blood Institute
National High Blood Pressure Education Program
120/80 National Institutes of Health
Bethesda, Maryland 20205

Arthritis Foundation
3400 Peachtree Road NE
Atlanta, Georgia 30326

American Diabetes Association
2 Park Avenue
New York, New York 10016

American Cancer Society
90 Park Avenue
New York, New York 10016

We have selected only a few major issues to discuss in this chapter; our survey indicated that hysterectomy and breast cancer were areas that women wanted discussed in detail. You can find general discussions of other female health issues in *Our Bodies, Ourselves: The AMA Guide to Womancare*; *MS. Guide to Woman's Health*; and *A New View of a Woman's Body*.

"If we feel good about ourselves and take things in stride as part of nature, I think life treats us better."

"I like the natural approach: vitamins, good diet, good attitude to tackling any symptoms. My mother had no problem, so I knew I'd do well."

"Knowing what decisions were made and why they were made has been important to me in dealing with menopause. Talking personally with people (women) I like and admire is also part of it. My choice(s) is not necessarily the one they made, but understanding the thought process and options open to them has helped me make decisions I will live with."

4

OSTEOPOROSIS: WHAT IT IS, WHO'S AT RISK, HOW IT'S DIAGNOSED

"Does it help to take the calcium supplements now, or is it too late for them to do any good?"

"I'm annoyed that my doctor has never offered any information on bone loss or osteoporosis. I became aware of the possible problem through TV and print ads for calcium supplements, also through magazine and newspaper articles, and just started taking calcium on my own."

"I'd like to see physicians' advice on preventing such problems as osteoporosis, whether good diet and exercise are adequate or food supplements are desirable."

"Do I take calcium supplements? No. Last year my doctor prescribed two TUMS a day, but then I developed what appeared to be a kidney stone, so I stopped."

- Did your mother, grandmothers, or sisters ever have a fractured hip?
- Do they (or did they) have osteoporosis?
- Do you have a thin, small frame?
- Are you fair-skinned?
- Are you near- or post-menopausal?
- Were your ovaries surgically removed?
- Does your diet include enough calcium?
- Do you exercise enough?
- How is your overall health?
- Do you smoke or drink alcohol?
- Do you take medications for other conditions?

How likely are *you* to develop osteoporosis? Your answers to the above questions can help you determine your chances. In this chapter, you'll learn why certain personal risk factors may indicate that you are a possible candidate for osteoporosis. You'll also read about how your bones are maintained and a little about their structure. You'll become familiar with the state-of-the-art in assessing bone loss. And you'll learn why osteoporosis is now a concern to midlife women, their families, doctors, employers, and insurance carriers.

In the next chapter, you'll learn more about how to prevent osteoporosis and its complications.

If you are over age 40 and are like the respondents in the Holt-Kahn research, you are concerned with the "weak bones" disease. Of the 967 respondents, 75.4% named osteoporosis as the menopause issue that concerned them most.

The questions respondents asked most frequently were:

- If my mother had osteoporosis, will I have it, too?
- Is there scientific evidence that estrogen replacement therapy or calcium supplements really prevent osteoporosis?
- Should I take estrogen replacement therapy to prevent osteoporosis?
- When is the time to start taking calcium supplements?

Should *you* be concerned about osteoporosis? The answer is a definite yes, because one out of four postmenopausal women will have it. Estimates are that half or more of all fractures among adults may be related to osteoporosis. Up to 33% of women and more than 17% of all men could experience a hip fracture by age 90 (Louis Avioli, *The Osteoporotic Syndrome: Detection and Prevention* [Orlando, Fla.: Grune and Stratton, 1983]).

WHAT IS OSTEOPOROSIS?

Osteoporosis is a condition in which the bones become fragile because there is a decrease in skeletal mass and mineral density. In an individual with osteoporosis, a fall, blow, or even a stressful lifting action can cause one or more bones to fracture. The ones most often affected are the hip and spinal bones.

Osteoporosis is the most common of the diseases that affect bones. According to Stephen M. Krane, M.D. ("Disorders of Bone Formation and Resorption," *Scientific American*, September 1984) osteoporosis is the most significant underlying cause of skeletal fractures in late middle-aged and elderly women.

We all know older women who have a "dowager's hump," who seem to stoop over and shrink more with age, and who require hospitalization for a hip fracture after a minor fall. Many of these problems can be prevented.

WHAT HAPPENS TO YOUR BONES AS YOU AGE?

Osteoporosis is a slow-moving disease. Like high blood pressure, it is silent. It results from loss of bone and minerals over a period of years. Although bones may appear to be the same size, they become "thinned out" from ongoing loss of calcium and protein.

Not all of your bones are alike. They come in all sizes and shapes, and each is made of two *types* of bone:

- Cortical(compact)
- Trabecular (spongy)

Both types of bone contain calcium and protein.

Cortical (compact) bone, on the outer part of bones, looks solid and hard, and accounts for 80% of your entire skeleton. Compact bone mass increases during childhood and adolescence to a maximum level during the

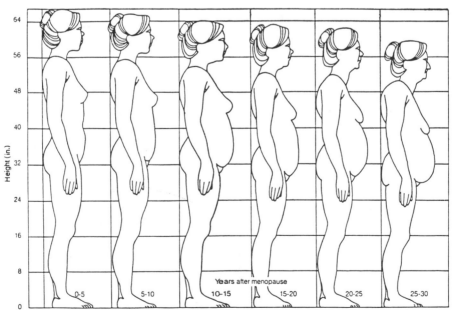

This chart shows the effects of osteoporosis in the years following menopause.
(A. A. Albanese, E. J. Lorenze, and E. H. Wein, *American Family Physician,* October 1978.)

thirties. The level remains stable for about 20 years and then declines. In postmenopausal women, loss accelerates.

Trabecular (spongy) bone, on the inside of bones, is filled with a honeycombed, spongelike material, and accounts for about 70% of your vertebral spine, hip bone, and intertrochanteric proximal femur (the "ball" of the hip). As you age, the walls of your compact bone become thinner and the holes in the spongy bone enlarge. Spongy bone mass increases until the thirties and from then on, there is a steady loss of bone in women (and in men, as well). The spinal bones, the hips, and the wrists have large amounts of spongy bone, and thus usually are the first targets for osteoporosis.

Within your bones, cells carry on three important processes:

- *Modeling* Bones develop into characteristic shapes.
- *Fracture repair* Damaged bones remove and replace themselves with new tissue and harden again.
- *Remodeling* The cells break down old bone and make new bone. Areas of bone dissolve and are absorbed back into the body.

Several personal factors interact to influence your bone-remodeling process:

- Genetic background, including race and sex.
- Exercise, particularly weight-bearing exercise.
- Nutrition, particularly your calcium intake.
- Endocrine status (Steroid hormones decrease and estrogens seem to help maintain bone mass. Parathyroid disorders may precipitate loss.) Certain adrenal disorders or administration of steroid drugs (cortisone, prednisone) on a chronic basis may increase bone loss.)

Your individual bone remodeling process affects your chances of getting osteoporosis. This process replaces about 8 to 12% of your bone mass each year. Until you reached adulthood, your body developed bone faster than it broke it down. You reached your peak bone mass around age 35 to 40.

Generally after age 35, the bone-remodeling process begins to reverse and bone breaks down and resorbs itself faster than new bone formation occurs, resulting in bone loss. The net loss in bone mass in both sexes is about 0.3% a year. The average woman from age 20 to 50 may lose more, about one-half to one per-cent per year.

However, immediately after menopause, the rate of bone loss accelerates. Studies report postmenopausal whole-skeleton bone loss rates as high as 2.5 to 3% per year. This rapid rate of loss slows down within a few years after menopause, and by the age of 70 to 75, women seem to lose bone mass at the same rate as men of comparable age (about 1 to 2% per year).

WHAT ARE THE SIGNS OF OSTEOPOROSIS?

Osteoporosis may go on for 15 to 20 years before a woman becomes aware that she has it. The first symptoms may be general back tiredness, back pain, or tenderness. Later, there may be a slight loss of height and a slight curvature of the upper back.

The most visible sign of well-established osteoporosis is "dowager's hump," a permanent curvature of the upper back. This happens when the spongy parts of the spinal bones become weakened under the weight of the upper body.

Other obvious signs of advanced osteoporosis are fractures, pain, deformity, and their consequences. Fractures happen most frequently in the hip and mid- and lower-thoracic and lumbar spine (the "small" of the back). Mild injury may cause fracture of the ball of the hip. Fractures of vertebrae may result from seemingly unlikely stress such as lifting, jumping, or even riding in a car on a bumpy road.

WHO IS MOST AT RISK?

There are some general clues in identifying women with low bone mass:

- Thin, white women, who have a low calcium intake, who have not had any children.
- Women who smoke.
- Short women, under 5'2", who weigh between 90 to 105 pounds—they have less bone mass than larger women and hence may fracture at a younger age if they lose bone.
- Black women have relatively little risk of bone loss. Osteoporotic fractures among black women are relatively rare.

According to the American College of Obstetricians and Gynecologists, the risk of osteoporosis after age 45 is higher in women than in men and in whites than in blacks. About nine times more women have osteoporosis than men. Twice as many elderly women as men are hospitalized or placed in nursing homes as a result of disabling fractures.

When any bone loss occurs in a small woman, a proportionally large part of her total bone mass is lost. Small, thin women have less fat tissue and therefore less estrogen, since fatty tissue chemically converts naturally occurring androgens to estrogen, even after the ovaries stop producing estrogen.

White women seem to develop osteoporosis more than black women because blacks generally have greater bone mass at maturity than whites. For similar reasons, women whose ancestors were from the British Isles, northern Europe, China, or Japan are more likely to get osteoporosis than those of African or Mediterranean ancestry.

Why this happens isn't clear, but it seems that some groups are characteristically smaller-boned than others, that osteoporosis runs in families, and that dietary habits may affect certain groups. However, there is no specific chromosomal problem known to lead to osteoporosis.

WHY DO MORE WOMEN THAN MEN GET OSTEOPOROSIS?

- Women are generally smaller-boned or lighter-boned
- Women's estrogen production tapers off after menopause
- Women may have less lifelong dietary calcium
- Women live longer than men (statistically)

Around the time of menopause, the ovaries cease producing estrogen; with less estrogen circulating in the body, the rate of bone loss increases. Especially in the few years just after menopause, a woman loses bone faster than a man of comparable age. There is a period of 3 to 5 years of rapid bone loss, then the rate of loss slows down over the next 5 to 10 years.

Physicians say that middle-aged and older women have less calcium in their diets than men, and that perhaps some women have been calcium-deficient all their lives. Perhaps this is because women are more likely than men to have followed weight loss diets that did not include adequate calcium.

Opinions differ on the effects of childbearing on osteoporosis. For example, according to the American College of Obstetricians and Gynecologists, some women may have greater calcium deficiencies than men because during pregnancy and breast-feeding, many women do not increase their intake of calcium to cover increased needs.

One study of women in nursing homes suggested that previous pregnancy had a protective effect. Some researchers have said that some women's bones were actually strengthened while they were subjected to more weight-bearing during the pregnancies.

According to Robert W. Cali, M.D., writing in *Postgraduate Medicine* (March 1984), "Pregnancy results in accumulation of maternal bone mass in excess of fetal needs. Multiparity [more than one pregnancy] can protect against osteoporosis."

Another factor may be that women who have had several children eat a better diet than women who have no children because, since they prepare nutritionally sound meals for their families, they also do so for themselves.

HOW IS BONE LOSS DETERMINED?

During an office visit, ask your physician about your chances for developing osteoporosis. Your physician will examine you and decide if you should have an evaluation for bone loss. You may be referred to a medical center or specialized osteoporosis center where diagnostic procedures can be performed.

There are several ways to determine rate of bone loss. X ray is a well-established method. Newer techniques are computerized axial tomography (CAT) scans and photon densitometry or photon absorptiometry studies. Biopsy is used only in special circumstances. In order to be an ideal screen for osteoporosis, a test would have to be inexpensive, accurate, easy to perform, readily available, and good at picking up early disease. At this time, no method meets these requirements, since most of the more accurate tests are expensive and not covered by insurance.

X ray (radiogrammetry)

X ray has been used as a diagnostic technique for osteoporosis for many years. Available since the 1950s, it is less widely used now that newer techniques are available

Advantages

- Can be done in some physicians' offices and in many radiology departments; widely available
- Is not invasive or uncomfortable for the patient
- As a research tool, the X ray techniques include measuring the width of a bone in the wrist with a caliper and the diameter or cortical thickness on X ray film
- X ray will reveal the width of the cortex of bone versus marrow cavity

Disadvantages

- X ray can reveal that osteoporosis is present, but not tell how much damage has been done to the bones.
- X rays have limited sensitivity; they measure mostly cortical bone loss. In some individuals, the major part of bone loss may be trabecular, particularly in the years after menopause.

Another disadvantage of X ray is that it may not be very useful in helping the physician recognize when an individual has less bone than considered standard for her age. Because of this deficiency, efforts have been made to develop more accurate techniques to measure bone mass as well as bone loss, and to compare them with pre-set standards.

More advanced bone mineral measurement techniques are available for clinical diagnosis, monitoring, and mass screening. Physicians now can evaluate a patient's bone mass and obtain subsequent information on bone changes with noninvasive techniques. Careful diagnosis depends on accurate measurement of fracture-sensitive areas, such as the lower spine and the hip joint. Measurement values are compared to a set of norms so that abnormalities may be detected.

Computerized Axial Tomography (CAT Scan)

Computerized axial tomography (CAT scan) measures bone mineral mass in a noninvasive way. It can measure the density of the trabecular (spongy) bone of the portion of the lumbar spine that is most susceptible to the effects of osteoporosis. The scan uses X rays of the bone taken at many different angles in order to visualize its internal structure. The average density of the bone is compared with data on standard density that are scanned along with each patient.

Advantages

- Measures trabecular (spongy bone) and a limited amount of cortical bone
- Machines are available in many medical centers
- Useful to assess early risk
- Useful to diagnose osteoporosis
- Useful to monitor a patient's course with osteoporosis

Disadvantages

- Knowing what the norms are. "They vary between geographic areas, even in the United States. We don't know why," says Robert Marcus, M.D., Director, Aging Study Unit, Veterans Administration Medical Center, Palo Alto, California, and Associate Professor of Medicine, Stanford University School of Medicine.
- Does not detect very early bone loss. When a woman has two sequential readings one year apart, the diagnostician can tell the rate of bone loss, but one year is lost before any treatment is initiated.
- Expensive.

- Relatively large dose of radiation. Computerized axial tomography of the vertebral spine gives a radiation exposure of at least 200 millirem, and as much as 1,500 millirem, considerably more than other techniques.
- Accuracy depends on proper patient positioning and composition of the bone marrow.
- Procedure can be intimidating and uncomfortable.

Photon Absorptiometry or Densitometry

Single photon absorptiometry

This technique was developed during the mid-1960s to measure compact bone of the arms, hands, legs, and feet.

In this procedure, a woman typically places her forearm (the distal radius or the wrist) between a beam of low-level radiation and a detector.

Although theoretically any peripheral bone can be measured, the most widely studied ones are the radius and/or ulna of the arm. The most precise measurements are obtained when the same site is scanned repeatedly in different positions.

Advantages

- Detects early decrease in bone mass before the loss shows on X rays. When abnormalities are detected at early ages, such as 30 to 50, intervention may prevent them from getting worse.
- Radiation exposure is minuscule.
- Considered useful as a screening technique and to observe sequential changes in women known to have osteoporosis.
- Noninvasive and painless.

Disadvantages

- Single photon absorptiometry is most useful for measuring cortical (compact) bone and only a limited amount of trabecular (spongy) bone in which most osteoporosis occurs
- The spine and proximal femur (ball of the hip), two areas susceptable to the effects of osteoporosis, cannot be measured this way
- These machines are not widely used yet (although they may be more available than CAT)
- Fairly expensive (the cost per procedure is about $50 to $150, depending on where it is done); most effective if used for several years to calculate rate of loss

- Has not been in use for very long; therefore, it is unknown how well studies done at age 50 correlate with later disease.

Dual Photon Absorptiometry (DPA) or Dual Photon Densitometry

A more recently developed technique is dual photon absorptiometry (DPA). The technique is an improvement over single photon absorptiometry because it is useful for examining the spine and hips.

Reported advancements in this technique led the American College of Physicians to select DPA over CAT as the preferred method of assessing bone disease, as reported in the *Annals of Internal Medicine* (June 1984). The National Institutes of Health also added their support for DPA as the preferred method at their 1984 Consensus Conference as reported in the *Journal of the American Medical Association* (August 1984).

The technique is somewhat like single photon absorptiometry, except that with DPA, the radiation beam moves back and forth over the patient as she lies on a table, and the amount of radiation that passes through her lower spine or hip joint is measured.

Advantages

- Measures bone mineral loss in lower spine and hip joint, where osteoporosis is most devastating
- Is not invasive or uncomfortable to patient
- Takes only 15 to 20 minutes for a lower spine or hip joint examination
- Useful both for initial diagnosing of abnormalities and for monitoring changes in the condition
- Cost, while more than that for an X ray, is generally about half the cost of a CAT scan
- Radiation exposure from the dual photon technique is up to 300 times lower (about 5 to 30 millirem versus 500 to 1500 millirem) than that of a CAT examination

Disadvantages

- Relatively expensive. Cost to the patient is typically about $100 to $250 per exam. May be but is not always covered by private health insurance carriers.
- Cost makes the procedure too expensive for mass screening.
- Same long-term questions as with single photon studies.

Should you ask for a bone densitometry study?

"Testing for bone loss can give someone who is worried a number to think about. If her bone mass is found to be low, she will pay more attention to her calcium intake," says Dr. Marcus. "And, of course, it is an excellent way to diagnose an early case of osteoporosis."

Although dual photon absorptiometry equipment is becoming more widely available, at this time the procedures are not used often in clinical practice. "It is hard to say when a woman should ask for this procedure," says Dr. Marcus:

> The average doctor doesn't yet have guidelines about how or when to do it. My preference is to screen large numbers of women. If we see evidence of deficiency, we check the woman again to determine changes. If there are changes, we may give her calcium supplements. We look at her metabolic rate, physiology, and hormonal status. Depending on her age and physical health, we might start estrogen replacement.

Other researchers and clinicians agree that screening procedures are important in preventing complications of osteoporosis. However, Richard B. Mazess, Ph.D., Department of Medical Physics, University of Wisconsin, says that in screening, only 5% of women show abnormalities as opposed to 50% when the methods are used only for women who have a specific indication for the test.

"The magnitude of the problems generated by post-menopausal osteoporosis is so great that we should make more efforts at prevention. As methods are improved to study bone density, we will use bone vertebral density just as we currently use mammography," says Will G. Ryan, M.D., Director, Osteoporosis Center, Rush-Presbyterian-St. Luke's Medical Center, Chicago. "Osteoporosis is a silent disease until it is too late. Like high blood pressure, it is more cost-effective to measure for it and do something about it than wait for its effects."

Biopsy

Bone biopsy involves removing a small piece of bone for study.

Advantages

- May help in the diagnosis for some premenopausal women who have clinical signs resembling those of postmenopausal osteoporosis
- May help in diagnosis when there is suspicion of osteomalacia or bone cancer

Disadvantages

- Invasive and painful
- Expensive

Other Tests Still in the Research Stage

Biochemical evaluations

Researchers are trying to find biochemical tests for bone loss. For example, increase in urinary free cortisol and a reduction of progesterone are associated with more rapid bone loss. Specifics under investigation include:

- Measurement of urinary free cortisol
- Measurement of progesterone
- Various bone proteins
- Urinary calcium

These and other research procedures, including neutron activation, have limited clinical use.

WHY BE CONCERNED ABOUT OSTEOPOROSIS?

Osteoporosis and hip fractures used to be considered merely "old women's issues." Now, according to the National Institute of Arthritis, Diabetes, and Digestive and Kidney Diseases, at least 15 million Americans have some degree of osteoporosis. Osteoporosis is directly linked to more than 150,000 hip fractures each year, according to a study conducted at the Mayo Clinic in Rochester, Minnesota. About 15% of all women with hip fractures die within three months because of such complications as pneumonia, blood clots, and stroke due to immobilization. Costs of caring for hip fractures in the United States, in 1990, are estimated to be more than triple what they were in 1965. Survivors require much care and many need prosthetic hips. Hip fractures cost health insurers billions of dollars a year. As more women live longer, the number of women who have brittle, weak bones increases. Thus osteoporosis has become a national problem.

You have seen in this chapter that osteoporosis *can* be detected in its early stages. Diagnostic techniques now can measure bone loss over a period of years.

Diagnostic tests for osteoporosis will become less expensive as technology develops, and eventually will be covered by more health insurers as there is increasing evidence that diagnosing osteoporosis in the early stages is less expensive in the long run than paying for the treatment of so many hip fractures and their complications.

Now that you see the magnitude of the problem of osteoporosis, what can you do to protect yourself—and your daughters?

In the following chapter, you'll find many helpful suggestions.

5
OSTEOPOROSIS: PREVENTION AND TREATMENT

There are many steps you can take to protect yourself—and your daughters—against osteoporosis. These steps are safe and sure for most women. And while protecting against osteoporosis, you may also improve your overall health.

- Exercise regularly
- Maintain your weight at a near-ideal level
- Include a balance of vitamins and minerals in your diet
- Include adequate dietary calcium (Young adults: 1,000 mg/day) (After menopause: 1,500 mg/day)
- Avoid excessive alcohol and caffeine
- Don't smoke

There are many aspects to successful, graceful aging. To maintain strong bones, there has to be a delicate balance between your level of exercise and your nutrition. You may reduce your chances of developing osteoporosis by changing several factors, including improving your diet, maintaining appropriate weight, exercising more, avoiding excessive intake of caffeine and alcohol, and not smoking. All these aspects of daily living interact to contribute to your overall good health and strong bone structure.

Smoking is an important factor in menopause. Menopause seems to occur two and one-half to three years earlier in women who smoke, and osteoporosis seems to affect more women whose menopause occurred early.

There are additional steps you can take; a few of these are currently somewhat controversial, and the controversies will be explained in this chapter.

- Consider taking calcium supplements.
- Consider taking estrogen replacement therapy after your physician carefully evaluates your personal risk-benefit tradeoff. (You'll also read more details about overall advantages and disadvantages of estrogen replacement therapy in the next chapter.)
- Consider obtaining an evaluation of the status of your bone mass by one of several recently developed diagnostic techniques (described in the previous chapter).

ROLE OF EXERCISE THROUGHOUT LIFE

A high level of physical activity throughout life can result in increased skeletal mass during the forties and fifties, when a large reservoir of bone mass may help delay symptoms of osteoporosis. Medical studies indicate that physical activity retards or prevents bone loss in recently postmenopausal as well as elderly women.

"There is little preventive medicine in the field of orthopedics," says Donald A. Nagel, M.D., Professor and Head, Division of Orthopedic Surgery, Stanford University School of Medicine. "Keep moving, that's the preventive medicine I preach." Dr. Nagel calls attention to the fact that in a study of 70 professional tennis players, bones were twice as thick on the athletes' playing side as on the other side.

Dr. Nagel advises doing-weight bearing exercises throughout life. Examples of weight-bearing exercises are walking, running, rope jumping, and aerobic dancing. Swimming is *not* weight bearing. While not useful to the skeleton, it is good for muscles, particularly those of the upper body.

Weight-bearing exercise is important because it puts stress on bones and induces chemical or electrical signals to pass to cells in bone and cause them to work more efficiently. Some degree of bone forms and retains calcium. "Because bone is in a continual process of breakdown and renewal, you can actually stimulate renewal by putting stress on your bones. You can accumulate bone mass with exercise," says Dr. Nagel. "There can be a reversal of *early* osteoporosis. Bones heal and thicken. Bone can gain ability to bear weight."

Several researchers have documented that endurance training in preparation for a marathon increases bone mass, and that middle-aged women can increase skeletal mass with modest weight-bearing programs. Even elderly individuals can improve their bones with mild weight-bearing exercise.

The effects of lack of weight-bearing exercise have been known to physicians for a long time. For example, children with paralysis due to paralytic polio develop hypercalciuria, (excess calcium in urine), hypercalcemia (excess calcium in blood stream), and bone loss. Bed rest for even a few weeks can lead to a loss of trabecular (spongy) bone mass. In recent years, mild bone losses have been noticed in astronauts who have spent time in weightless orbit.

It is possible to overexercise however. "Too much exercise puts an increased load on the heart," says Dr. Nagel. Also, "in our specialized medical center, we see many patients with overuse syndromes such as stress fractures of the pelvis, or femur, who have been referred by other physicians. These patients have actually injured their bones by putting too much stress on them."

Too much exercise can also *cause* osteoporosis. "Some women athletes who regularly run more than 10 miles a day or do other strenuous exercise may be predisposed to bone loss if they stop ovulating and menstruating. Observations have been made that such women have less bone than some non-exercising women their age," says Gregory R. Mundy, M.D., Head, Division of Endocrinology and Metabolism, Department of Medicine, University of Texas Health Science Center, San Antonio, Texas. "However, bone loss in these athletic women is reversible. If they cut down on strenuous activity, menstruation will occur again. I urge exercise in *moderation* for most women."

MAINTAIN NEAR-IDEAL WEIGHT WITH A WELL-BALANCED DIET

Rapid weight losses and gains may take a toll on your body. Being too thin or too heavy for your age and body build may put extra stresses on all your vital organs and body systems. To maintain your weight at a near-ideal level, eat a well-balanced diet. Women over age 45 should be particularly careful to include adequate calcium and Vitamin D, as well as enough other essential vitamins and minerals. (See chapter 8 for more details.)

Importance of Dietary Calcium

Calcium, the most abundant mineral in your body, accounts for about 1.5 to 2% of your total body weight. Calcium is distributed throughout bone and teeth (99%) and in blood, body fluids, and various soft tissues (1%).

Calcium is critical for effective cardiac, nerve, and muscle function, and to impart strength to bones and teeth.

Without appropriate calcium intake, exercise is not as useful for maintaining bone structure. If calcium is not available from outside sources, the only resource is bone, and when calcium is taken from the bones over a period of years, the supportive structure of the skeleton is weakened.

FOODS HIGH IN CALCIUM
(More Than 25 Milligrams Calcium per Serving)

Food	Approximate amount	Weight gm	Calcium mg
Meat Group			
Egg	1	50	27
Fish			
Salmon (with bones)	1 oz	30	51
Sardines	1 oz	30	115
Clams	1 oz	30	29
Oysters	1 oz	30	31
Shrimp	1 oz	30	35
Cheese			
Cheddar	1 oz	30	218
Cheese foods	1 oz	30	160
Cheese spread	1 oz	30	158
Cottage cheese	1/4 cup	50	53
Fat			
Cream			
Half and half	2 T	30	32
Sour	2 T	30	31
Bread Group			
Bread			
Biscuit	2″ diameter	35	42
Muffin	2″ diameter	35	36
Cornbread	1 1/2 cube	35	36
Pancake	4″ diameter	45	45
Waffle	1/2 square	35	39
Beans, dry (canned or cooked)	1/2 cup	90	45
Lima beans	1/2 cup	100	42
Parsnips	2/3 cup	100	45
Milk			
Whole	1 cup	240	288
Evaporated whole milk	1/2 cup	120	302
Powdered whole milk	1/2 cup	30	252
Buttermilk	1 cup	240	296
Skim milk	1 cup	240	298
Powdered skim milk, dry	1/4 cup	30	367
Fruit			
Blackberries	3/4 cup	100	32
Orange	1 medium	100	41
Raspberries	3/4 cup	100	30
Rhubarb	1 cup	100	96
Tangerine	2 small	100	40

(cont. on next page)

FOODS HIGH IN CALCIUM (Continued)

Food	Approximate amount	Weight gm	Calcium mg
Vegetable A, cooked			
Beans, green or wax	1/2 cup	100	50
Beet greens	1/2 cup	100	99
Broccoli	1/2 cup	100	88
Cabbage	1/2 cup	100	49
Cabbage, Chinese	1/2 cup	100	43
Celery	1/2 cup	100	39
Chard	1/2 cup	100	73
Collards	1/2 cup	100	188
Cress	1/2 cup	100	81
Dandelion greens	1/2 cup	100	140
Mustard greens	1/2 cup	100	138
Sauerkraut	1/2 cup	100	36
Spinach	1/2 cup	100	93
Squash, summer	1/2 cup	100	25
Turnip greens	1/2 cup	100	184
Turnips	1/2 cup	100	35
Vegetable B, cooked			
Artichokes	1/2 cup	100	51
Brussels sprouts	1/2 cup	100	32
Carrots	1/2 cup	100	33
Kale	1/2 cup	100	187
Kohlrabi	1/2 cup	100	33
Leeks, raw	3-4	100	52
Okra	1/2 cup	100	92
Pumpkin	1/2 cup	100	25
Rutabagas	1/2 cup	100	59
Squash, winter	1/2 cup	100	28
Dessert			
Cake, white	1 piece	50	32
Custard, baked	1/3 cup	100	112
Ice cream	1/2 cup	75	110
Ice milk	1/2 cup	75	118
Pie, cream	1/6 of 9″ pie	160	120
Pudding	1/2 cup	100	117
Sherbet	1/3 cup	50	25

Note: This chart is reproduced from *Food, Nutrition and Diet Therapy* by M. V. Krause and M. A. Hunscher. Philadelphia: W. B. Saunders Co., 1972.

From *Mayo Clinic Diet Manual,* 4th Ed. Philadelphia: W. B. Saunders Co., 1971.

Not all authorities agree on how much calcium is necessary. For example, the Recommended Dietary Allowance (RDA) requirements for calcium in postmenopausal women are too low, according to Dr. Robert Marcus of Stanford Medical Center.

A report in the February 1985 *Journal of Clinical Nutrition* indicated that whereas the generally accepted RDA for calcium of 800 milligrams (mg) was probably adequate for young adults, it grossly underestimated the needs of postmenopausal women, which are closer to 1,500 mg/day.

Robert Recker, M.D. and Robert Heaney, M.D. of the Creighton University School of Medicine reported that postmenopausal women require 1,500 mg calcium/day to achieve calcium balance. (Calcium balance is the difference between calcium consumed in the diet and that excreted in feces, sweat and urine. The ideal balance is zero.)

"Calcium is the basis for protection against osteoporosis. Maximize calcium," emphasizes Dr. Licata of the Cleveland Clinic. He advises a daily intake of one gram per day before menopause. "The requirement rises over 50% after menopause," he says.

Why more calcium is needed after menopause seems to be related to alterations in Vitamin D levels or intestinal malabsorption as we age. With increasing age, for unknown reasons, the ability of our intestine to absorb and of our kidneys to retain calcium decreases.

Milk as a source of calcium

"The simplest source is milk, either as whole or skim milk, or yogurt," advises Dr. Marcus. "After menopause, women need the equivalent of one and one-half quarts each day," he says.

To build strong bones, we should encourage calcium intake before menopause. Encourage your daughters and younger sisters to drink more milk before menopause! Even after menopause, drinking milk can be helpful in preventing the onset or development of osteoporosis. However, many adults develop cramps and bloating when they ingest this much milk. See the following suggestions. Also, you should keep your fat intake as low as possible, so skim milk and low-fat cheeses are best.

Other food sources

Other dairy foods, such as yogurt and ice cream, are also excellent sources of calcium. Surprisingly, one cup of low-fat yogurt contains more calcium than the same amount of milk. Dairy products are good sources of calcium because of their high calcium content and, more importantly, because the calcium is readily available for absorption. Nutrients in milk and other dairy foods, such as lactase and Vitamin D, favor calcium absorption.

Certain meat group foods, such as canned sardines and salmon containing soft, edible bones, have a high calcium content. You can get the equivalent of one cup of milk by eating one and a half ounces of sardines or five ounces of canned red salmon. Other calcium-rich foods are shellfish, almonds, brazil nuts, dried beans, and soybean curd (tofu).

Broccoli, kale, bok choy, collards, and the greens of turnip, mustard, and dandelion are also good sources of calcium.

How you cook your foods can make a difference in the amount of calcium you derive from them. For example, cooking meat or fish bones leaches calcium from them, making the resulting broth a good source of dietary calcium. Add vegetables and you'll have a nutritious and tasty soup. You'll find more helpful hints on how to maximize the nutritional content of foods you prepare in chapter 8.

Choose dietary protein carefully to retain calcium

Protein in your diet also can help regulate your calcium balance. How much protein do you need? Dr. Marcus says 70 to 80 grams per day, and that most of us get 110 to 120 grams each day from our diet. Too much protein causes a negative calcium balance. He advises consuming more milk or meat foods for protein, because those foods lead to less calcium loss than when protein is derived from vegetables. However, protein foods should be chosen carefully to avoid high fat content.

"We can speculate what should be done. We'll know in 20 years if we are right. Most people have a lack of calcium. They have a 'snack and run' kind of lifestyle. They don't consume enough dairy products. Dietary deprivation of calcium in the growing years causes the bones to be less strong than they should be, says Dr. Licata. "In recent years, many young people seem to substitute soft drinks for milk."

Vitamin D and calcium absorption

Vitamin D is necessary to regulate your absorption of calcium. You get Vitamin D from the action of sunlight on your skin and from dietary sources. A Vitamin D deficiency makes intestinal absorption of calcium less efficient. As we age, we have a decreasing ability to manufacture Vitamin D, and thus less ability to absorb calcium. "It may be useful for the elderly to take 1,000 to 2,000 units of Vitamin D daily," says Dr. Marcus. However, too much Vitamin D can be toxic and even *promote* bone loss. The American Society for Bone and Mineral Research recommends that individuals not take more than 1,000 international units (IU) per day unless it is prescribed by a physician.

Taking Calcium Supplements

According to the American Society for Bone and Mineral Research, eating a well-balanced diet is the best way to ensure an adequate calcium intake. However, many women cannot consume enough milk and dairy products, and for them, calcium supplements may be necessary. (You'll read how women with a lactose intolerance deal with the problem of getting enough calcium in their diet in chapter 8.)

Results of the Holt-Kahn survey indicate that many women are taking calcium supplements in tablets, powder, and liquid. Of 967 respondents, 59.5% said they take calcium supplements; of those, 32.1% reported that their physicians prescribed the supplements, while 69.8 are taking them on a self-prescribed basis.

The advantages and disadvantages of each are summarized in the table below.

CALCIUM SUPPLEMENTS

Form	%Calcium	Comment
Calcium carbonate	40	Relatively insoluble. Not absorbed well in individuals who lack sufficient stomach acid. May cause constipation. Used in several antacids.
Calcium Chloride	36	Rarely given orally. May irritate the stomach.
Calcium Lactate	13	Contains relatively little calcium.
Calcium Gluconate	9	Very little calcium.
Bone Meal	31	Also contains phosphorus, sodium, magnesium, potassium, sulphur, copper, and iodine. May be contaminated with toxic metals such as arsenic, mercury, lead, cadmium, and others.
Dolomite	22	Also contains magnesium, chloride, iron, and phosphorus. May be contaminated with toxic metals such as arsenic, mercury, lead, cadmium, and others. Major ingredient in several antacids.

Source: *Calcium: A Summary of Current Research for the Health Professional,*
Courtesy National Dairy Council.

Many women seem to know that taking five TUMS a day provides about 2.5 grams (that's 2,500 milligrams) of calcium carbonate, which is 40% calcium. In fact, many physicians seem to advise their "worried well" patients who think they should be taking calcium supplements to take TUMS.

Of all calcium supplements available, calcium carbonate has the most calcium per gram.

Some gastric acidity is necessary to dissolve TUMS; therefore, they may be less useful for women who take acid secretion inhibitors.

However, research reported in the *New England Journal of Medicine* indicates that when calcium carbonate is taken *with meals*, it is well absorbed even in women without endogenous gastric acidity. For most women who take calcium supplements, the Dairy Nutrition Council recommends that they be taken between meals or at different times throughout the day. You can increase your calcium absorption by taking the supplement with a small amount of milk or yogurt; both contain Vitamin D and lactose, which encourage calcium absorption.

Women who self-prescribe their calcium supplements should be careful. Excessive calcium has also been linked to kidney stones; therefore it is a good idea to discuss with your doctor the best form and dose of calcium for you. Additionally, be careful about self-prescribing dolomite or bone meal as a calcium supplement because there is published evidence that severe neurological damage due to lead can result from prolonged consumption of bone meal, most likely due to contaminants such as lead or arsenic.

While there is popular belief that other minerals are necessary to properly absorb calcium, there is some disagreement about why this may be so, if it is so. Dr. Marcus says: "There's no evidence that a calcium supplement must be taken along with extra minerals of any other sort." Dr. Licata says: "Magnesium is also important, and is involved in maintaining normal levels of calcium in the blood. However, there is insufficient evidence that supplementary magnesium does anything to preserve the calcium in bone. The role of zinc is unknown.

"The role of phosphorus is important, but too much can have an adverse effect. A higher proportion of phosphorus to calcium may be harmful. (Phosphorus-rich foods include meat and soft drinks.) In animals, large doses of phosphorus have been known to cause osteoporosis."

Some women should NOT take calcium supplements

Uriel Barzel, M.D., Professor of Medicine, Albert Einstein College of Medicine, Bronx, New York, warns that women who have kidney stones (calcium stones) or hyperparathyroidism should *not* take calcium supplements.

Role of Sodium Fluoride and Osteoporosis

Results of recent studies from the Mayo Clinic suggest that fluoride may have a role in the treatment of osteoporosis by reducing the risk of vertebral compression fractures.

Advantages

- Given with supplemental calcium and Vitamin D, sodium fluoride may decrease bone resorption.

- Given in a dosage of 1 milligram/kilogram of weight, it may stimulate bone formation and increase trabecular bone mass.
- When used in combination with estrogen, it may make new fractures less likely.

Disadvantages

- High toxicity level.
- Side effects include gastrointestinal irritation and vomiting; also anemia and arthritic pains (Scientific American, Inc., 1984).
- At this time, no fluoride preparation has been approved by the U.S. Food and Drug Administration for treatment of osteoporosis. Studies are under way under the auspices of the National Institutes of Health. Treatment with fluoride should be performed only at facilities with appropriate equipment to monitor all aspects of fluoride treatment.

Phosphate Supplements and Osteoporosis

Some researchers (Stephen M. Krane, M.D., "Disorders of Bone Formation and Resorption," *Scientific American*, September 1984) advocate phosphate supplements to improve calcium balance by decreasing urinary calcium excretion. This is *highly* controversial because high phosphate intake may be a *cause* of osteoporosis in some individuals.

ROLE OF HORMONES IN OSTEOPOROSIS

Estrogen first was suggested as a preventive or treatment for osteoporosis about 45 years ago. The therapy lost favor, but in recent years has gained many adherents, due to new research about its effectiveness and safer ways of using ERT.

Estrogen replacement therapy (ERT) is also used to treat other symptoms of menopause and postmenopause. You'll read more about the overall advantages and disadvantages of ERT in chapter 6. In this chapter, we'll show why one's own reduced estrogen supply leads to bone loss and how ERT may contribute to maintenance of postmenopausal bone mass.

After menopause, reduction of the body's own estrogen and progesterone seems to accelerate bone loss in many women who develop bone problems. There are varying opinions among physicians and researchers regarding use of estrogen replacement to halt bone loss. However, on balance, more literature points to estrogen replacement therapy as being helpful as an osteoporosis preventive.

Numerous studies have shown that estrogen replacement conserves skeletal mass and protects against fractures. One study was reported in the *Annals of Internal Medicine* in March 1985 in which fractures in long-term estrogen users were compared with case-matched controls over an average 17.6 year period. Researchers Ettinger, Genant, and Cann said that results of the study suggested that long-term estrogen replacement therapy does give significant protection against bone loss and fracture. In this study, quantitative bone mineral assessments were obtained from 18 women who used estrogen replacement therapy and a similar number not using estrogen replacement therapy. The women averaged 73 years old. There were half as many osteoporotic fractures among the estrogen users as among the control group. Estrogen users showed 54.2% greater spinal mineral and 19.4% greater forearm mineral.

Some physicians believe that the time to intervene with estrogen therapy is early, not later, because by the time "menopause" is obvious and the woman has ceased having menses for a year significant bone loss may have occured. "To maintain skeletal mass, the dose of estrogen also maintains menstrual periods. Many women after age 50 will elect to stop taking the estrogen on their own and also stop having resultant periods," says Dr. Marcus.

For those who take estrogen replacement therapy for osteoporosis, when should they stop? "There are implications that we can preserve bone indefinitely. Women would lose bone rapidly if they stopped taking estrogen, once they start," says Dr. Will Ryan of Rush-Presbyterian-St. Luke's Medical Center. "Combined with progestational agents (hormones which 'protect' the uterine lining and probably breasts from excessive estrogen), the incidence of cancer is greatly reduced—in fact, better than taking nothing at all. Endometrial cancer is overrated. The rate of death from endometrial cancer is less than 1%," he says. (You'll read more about the general advantages and disadvantages of estrogen replacement therapy in chapter 6.) Endometrial cancer is cancer of the uterine lining, linked to high-dose, continuous ERT.

Benefits of Estrogen Therapy for Preventing/Treating Osteoporosis

"The more miserable elderly women I see with osteoporosis, the more I think we should recommend estrogen therapy for all women," says Dr. Ryan. Dr. Ryan summarizes the benefits as outweighing the risks:

- Women on estrogen live longer; possibilities of fractures are reduced, thus reducing possible complications that might result in death.
- It tends to decrease incidence of cardiovascular disease.

- Combined with progestational agents, it may reduce the incidence of breast cancer.

However, not all women can take estrogen. You may have been advised against taking estrogen replacement if you have a history of blood clots, high blood pressure, any type of cancer, or any breast disease.

"Estrogen prevents the acceleration of bone loss, but we don't recommend estrogen for everyone because this would expose some women who may not need the drug to side effects. A person can have bone loss and no symptoms," says Dr. Licata.

Controversies within the medical profession

There is disagreement among the medical profession regarding estrogen replacement as a routine treatment or preventive for osteoporosis. One who does not favor routine use of estrogen replacement is Dr. Mundy:

> I would consider using it for a person who is particularly predisposed to development of osteoporosis later on, such as a Caucasian woman with early menopause, small stature, and a family history of the disease. Estrogen slows the accelerated bone resorption that occurs around the time of menopause, but I'm not convinced that it affects the universal, progressive, age-related bone loss, or that it is beneficial in women over age 60. If I started a woman on estrogen when she was 50, it is likely that I would recommend taking her off of it at age 60. There's no guarantee that anyone taking estrogen won't get osteoporosis and for some women, estrogen may be a cancer risk.

Dr. Mundy, like many physicians, prescribes estrogen only to women at high risk for osteoporosis, such as those who are slim, blonde, inactive, and who are cigarette-smokers who had early menopause.

"Nearly all cases of established osteoporosis are in people age 60 or older," he says. "These patients, mostly women, often have painful backs and fractures. Estrogen does nothing, I think, to prevent or relieve this. There's just no scientific evidence for it."

Regulation of estrogen dosage

For women who do take estrogen, the dose may have to be individualized. Estrogens are metabolized (broken down) in the liver. High alcohol intake causes the liver to metabolize estrogen faster. Certain medications (barbiturates used in seizure disorders and some tranquilizers) also speed the breakdown. These women may need a little more estrogen. Women with liver damage from alcohol abuse or hepatitis may need less. Very elderly women may need less.

New techniques are being developed to release constant small amounts of estrogen. These techniques may reduce some of the side effects of estrogen replacement therapy, such as nausea, bloating, and breast tenderness. You'll read more about new routes for drug administration later in this chapter.

Effects of Oral Contraceptives

For young women who are estrogen deficient, oral contraceptives can help maintain bone mass.

Effects of Androgen Derivatives

In controlled studies, androgen derivatives have been shown to increase bone mass. "However, androgen-related side effects constrain widespread use of this approach," says Dr. Marcus. Effects of androgen derivatives may be excess growth of body hair and voice changes.

What to Ask Your Doctor When Estrogen Is Prescribed for You to Prevent/Treat Osteoporosis

Dozens of respondents to the Holt-Kahn survey asked questions about perceived "hazards" of taking estrogen replacement therapy as an osteoporosis preventive/treatment. Each woman's physiology is unique, and rather than give generalizations here, we suggest that you discuss your personal situation with your physician. However, if you have any doubts about why you should start this therapy as a preventive/treatment for osteoporosis, here's what to ask:

- Am I far enough along in my menopausal course to start estrogen replacement?
- If my periods have not yet stopped, will taking estrogen to prevent osteoporosis also prolong my periods?
- What changes can I expect in my periods (longer, shorter, heavier, lighter)?
- Should I expect other physical changes, such as effects on my breasts?
- Am I too far past my menopause for estrogen replacement therapy to do me much good?
- If I haven't menstruated in 10 years, will taking estrogen cause periods to resume?

There's much more to the estrogen replacement story, as we see in chapter 6.

THOSE WHO HAVE OSTEOPOROSIS CAN MAKE THEIR LIVES EASIER

Be Safe, Not Sorry

Persons who have osteoporosis should take extra safety precautions to minimize the risk of falls. For example, wear appropriate shoes, place adequate lighting in hallways and stairways, and remove items over which you may trip. Be careful to use nonslip bathroom rugs, install grab bars on your tub and shower, and carpet stairs so they will not be slippery. Also, minimize the number of medications you take that might cause dizziness or confusion.

Women who have osteoporosis may benefit from research on products that make activities of daily living for arthritis sufferers easier. You may write to get a copy of the "Self Help Manual for Patients with Arthritis" from:

> The Arthritis Foundation
> 3400 Peachtree Road NE,
> Atlanta, Georgia 30326

Avoid Medications That May Aggravate Osteoporosis

"Certain diseases and their treatments will accelerate osteoporosis even in young people," says Dr. Mundy. He explains that anyone taking steroid drugs for more than six months may be at risk. "People who must take steroids for asthma, kidney disorders, forms of arthritis, and some other problems may develop osteoporosis. So do people with Cushing's Syndrome, a condition that causes the body to produce excessive steroids. These disorders simply wash out the bones in young people."

Dr. Mundy also says that by some unknown process, alcohol directly poisons new bone formation. Bones of alcoholics are more fragile than those of others. Cigarette smoking and excessive caffeine intake also harm new bone formation.

Various medications can affect the availability of calcium in the body. Several commonly used medications, such as isoniazid for the treatment of pulmonary tuberculosis, corticosteroids, the antibiotic tetracycline, and aluminum-containing antacids for treating acute peptic ulcers and gastritis, can increase the urinary calcium excretion, and, as such, accelerate bone loss, according to the National Dairy Council.

When and Where to Go for Help About Osteoporosis

"The first sign may be persistent back pain," says Dr. Licata. "Your back should be strong enough to enable you to stand for long periods of time. If you are more comfortable lying down, something is wrong and you should be checked over." However, low back pain can have many different causes, such as muscle strain, obesity, or a slipped disc.

Gynecology, endocrinology, and orthopedics are medical specialties that all take an interest in osteoporosis. The important thing is to go early for medical help. Find a physician familiar with osteoporosis. This could be an endocrinologist, rheumatologist, internist, family practitioner, or obstetrician-gynecologist.

Different physicians use different methods of diagnosing osteoporosis, depending on their facilities and equipment. At major medical centers or specialized osteoporosis centers, a woman may be evaluated with use of the dual photon technique. The rate of bone loss is determined only when two measurements using the same technique (maybe even the same machine) are done at two different times (usually at least a year apart).

In addition to evaluating bone loss by an imaging technique, blood tests for osteoporosis may be done. For example, from a sample of blood, the doctor would measure, among other things, calcium, phosphorus, pH (degree of alkalinity), phosphatase, albumin, globulin, creatinine, blood urea nitrogen, and liver function.

In many areas, some of the newer screening procedures are either unavailable or prohibitively expensive. Many insurance carriers do not cover "screening" procedures. In the near future the tests should be more available and affordable, and more insurance carriers may cover them.

If you go to a knowledgeable doctor's office, for the cost of an office visit, you may get a fair assessment based on your history of risk factors.

Osteoporosis centers may become increasingly common, just as free-standing emergency centers did during the early 1980s. For many women who have medical conditions which tend to lead to osteoporosis, and for those whose osteoporosis has been diagnosed, these centers will provide important sources of information and treatment. In 20 years, tests may be less expensive and women may have routine bone examinations as part of their complete medical screening.

WHAT'S AHEAD: CURRENT RESEARCH

Milk Versus Calcium Supplements

Calcium supplements and milk seem to have comparable benefits in retarding bone loss, although some researchers think milk may be absorbed better. Research currently in progress at the Creighton University School of Medicine may shed light on this question.

Relationship of Estrogen and Calcitonin

Researchers don't yet have clear ideas about how estrogen replacement therapy retards development of osteoporosis. One theory is that estrogen may affect calcitonin secretion; calcitonin inhibits bone resorption. The level of calcitonin goes down with age. However, calcitonin levels can be increased with estrogen treatment. When estrogen is withdrawn, there is less calcitonin present, and thus less inhibition of bone resorption.

Although controversial, a synthetic form of calcitonin is sometimes recommended for management of postmenopausal osteoporosis. The drug is given by injection three times per week and costs about $7 to $10 a day. The drug manufacturer recommends that calcitonin be given in conjunction with an adequate intake of Vitamin D and calcium.

There is disagreement among researchers regarding how calcitonin level affects osteoporosis. While early studies suggested that a calcitonin deficiency might be significant in the development of osteoporosis, in April 1985, researchers Robert D. Tiegs, M.D., et al., of the Mayo Clinic, Rochester, Minnesota, reported that serum calcitonin levels are *higher* than normal in postmenopausal women with untreated osteoporosis (*New England Journal of Medicine* 312 [April 25, 1985]: p. 1097). In 1984, results of research reported at the Copenhagen International Symposium on Osteoporosis reported that while calcitonin may slow the loss of bone mass, it has limited value in replacing bone previously lost. According to the *Medical Letter* (June 21, 1985), no studies have been published on long-term use of calcitonin in patients with postmenopausal osteoporosis.

Vitamin D Investigations

The active product of Vitamin D is being investigated for efficacy of treatment of postmenopausal osteoporosis. It may improve formation of new bone. Results of research findings are currently controversial. This agent must be used carefully. Too much may stimulate bone resorption.

New Routes for Drug Administration

Researchers also are looking at new ways to administer drugs for treatment of osteoporosis that will eliminate side effects and complications. For example, new routes of administration might have a protective effect on bones and arteries without inducing monthly bleeding (as may occur with administration of estrogen):

- *Estrogen administered through a patch worn on the skin.*
  Transdermal administration of estrogen may have an advantage

over estrogen taken orally because it allows direct absorption and seems to have less effect on blood levels of lipids and fatty acids. Orally, most of the estrogen goes through the liver and stimulates synthesis of proteins and coagulating factors that may result in blood clots. Additionally, in research studies, transdermal estrogen did not seem to increase the incidence of gallstones. (An overstressed liver is a major cause of gallstones.)

- *Development of a calcitonin product as a nasal spray.* This is in a research stage.

Calcium Citrate

- Research supported by a grant from the National Institute of Arthritis, Diabetes, and Digestive and Kidney Diseases at the University of Texas Health Sciences Center at Dallas focuses on use of calcium citrate supplementation. Results of preliminary studies by the researchers published in the August 1985 issue of the *Journal of Clinical Endocrinology and Metabolism* indicate that as a calcium supplement, calcium citrate is better absorbed through the walls of the intestine than calcium carbonate. Also, they report that calcium citrate supplementation has been shown to increase urinary citrate, a substance which inhibits formation of calcium stones.

SUMMARY

"Drink all of your milk to make your bones grow strong!"

"Stretch and bend to make your bones grow straight!"

Both are good reminders to prepare for a healthy menopause and life after menopause with strong and straight bones.

Tell your daughters to start while they are young to plan to be straight, healthy old ladies, because calcium intake affects bone structure at an early age. For some women the loss of bone density as a consequence of aging causes no problems. However, for all of us, preventing osteoporosis should be a lifelong goal.

Lifestyle changes to incorporate better diet, weight-bearing exercise, maintenance of weight at a near-ideal level, adequate intake of vitamins and minerals, low levels of caffeine and alcohol, and no smoking can help you protect yourself against osteoporosis.

Development of osteoporosis may be prevented, according to the 1984 National Institutes of Health Consensus Conference on Osteoporosis. However, the group cautioned against the potential complications of kidney stones from calcium supplementation in susceptible women. Also, osteoporosis can be detected in its earliest stages when it is somewhat treatable and complications can be avoided.

From a medical standpoint, there still is disagreement among experts about treatment. However, clinicians advocate estrogen replacement therapy for many women, despite possible risks. Enthusiasts of estrogen replacement therapy say it is more effective for the first five or six years past menopause. Also, supplemental calcium to prevent and treat osteoporosis is most effective in the early post menopausal years.

From a practical, self-help viewpoint, drinking milk and consuming other calcium-rich foods seems to make a difference. Physicians say that a lifelong consumption of large amounts of dietary calcium is like building up a large bank account. The equivalent of calcium bankruptcy is osteoporosis and fractures.

6

IS ESTROGEN REPLACEMENT THERAPY FOR YOU?

"It's not easy to be a well-informed menopausal woman these days. Keeping up with the latest medical information and recommendations about estrogen replacement therapy (ERT), a popular treatment for the symptoms of menopause, is a challenge even for experts in the field. Among those who stay on top of current research, there is widespread controversy over its inter- pretation."

Jane Brody, New York Times (April 17, 1985)

"Estrogen, it seems, may be one of those things some women can't live with and can't live without. . . . While some two million to three million postmenopausal women in the United States take estrogens daily, scientists are struggling to determine if the practice is ultimately helpful or harmful."

Science News 18 (November 1, 1985)

There is also controversy over estrogen replacement among our own respondents. Many agree that ERT can correct many menopausal symptoms, but many are also concerned that ERT has been associated with a number of potentially harmful or undesirable side effects. Of the 967 women who answered our question about taking hormones, 27% said they take them and 73% said they do not. Of interest is that 62% of the 52 gynecologists who responded to the same survey take them; 38% do not. Perhaps the women gynecologists know something the rest of us don't!

Here's what some women said about hormone replacement:

"There's much confusion about estrogen therapies. I wonder how many long- term studies there are with proven results about aftereffects?"

"I would rather not take pills, but estrogen-progesterone has made the quality of my life remarkably better. But still, in the back of my mind, I wonder if in the long run it could cause problems, such as cancer, although my gynecologist supports it with progesterone. I wonder how long I can safely stay on estrogen-progestogen therapy."

"ERT has been tried against my best judgment and caused me great problems—such as breakthrough bleeding."

"Now I wonder which form of hormone replacement is better and whether I have a choice."

"I'd like to see in your book reasons why to replace hormones; how to do it safely; and scientific information regarding menopause with and without supplement; who needs it, why, why not; in common language that is sound information. Also, when is it too late to do anything about hormones and osteoporosis?"

"I'd like to see the issue of early hysterectomy and its aftermath addressed with the issue of estrogen replacement in such cases."

"I would love to read some positive material about hormone pills, etc. Even though I'm on them because of my severe flashes, I'm scared to death of what they may do to me."

"I'd like to see a full discussion of hormone use, pros and cons. My ob-gyn and internist have differing opinions."

"What do you think about some doctors' suggestions that women take hormones the rest of their lives?"

"Address the issue of estrogen replacement and the customizing of same for each woman. We are not all alike!"

In this chapter you'll learn to develop your own benefit/risk profile, by finding out why ERT is prescribed for many women, what to ask your doctor if ERT is prescribed for you, advantages and disadvantages of therapy, what to ask if ERT is *not* prescribed for you, and what to consider if you can't take ERT.

The American College of Obstetricians and Gynecologists (ACOG) advises that not every woman can take estrogens. If you have had breast cancer or another type of cancer involving one of the reproductive organs, if you think you might be pregnant, if you have vaginal bleeding that is not a normal period, or if you have any disorder of blood clotting, talk with your doctor about other ways to deal with your symptoms of menopause, says the ACOG. You'll find more details about women who should not take estrogens later in this chapter.

SORTING OUT THE HORMONES

Hormones sometimes are prescribed to mimic or accentuate effects of the hormones that are naturally produced by the body. Most of the agents used therapeutically are either naturally occurring or synthetic chemical forms of naturally occurring hormones.

For menopausal and postmenopausal women, synthetic hormones are used to:

- Correct symptoms of hormonal imbalance, such as irregular bleeding
- Reverse an abnormal process, such as hirsutism or endometriosis
- Prevent and treat osteoporosis (see chapters 4 and 5)
- Treat hot flashes; make them less frequent and less severe
- Treat vaginal atrophy, irritation, itching, and burning
- Relieve some symptoms of painful sexual intercourse
- Somewhat relieve emotional changes experienced during menopause

In chapters 2 and 3 you read a little about the major "female" hormones, estrogens, and "male" hormones, androgens. Now here's some more information about how estrogens and related hormones affect your body throughout your life cycle. These details will help you understand why ERT can work for some women—but not for others—to relieve menopausal symptoms.

What Is Estrogen?

The *Oxford English Dictionary* defines estrogens as "sex hormones produced in the ovary usually characterized by ability to produce estrus and secondary sex characteristics in females."

The word estrogen is derived from the Greek *oistros* or Latin *oestrus* (meaning gadfly, frenzy, sexual heat, animal rut, desire) and the Greek suffix -*gen* (born, generate).

Estrogens are a diverse group of compounds. They include naturally occurring hormones that influence certain growth patterns, processes, and physical functions, and synthetic compounds with similar biologic properties. Estrogens are secreted and produced in different ways in premenopausal, perimenopausal and postmenopausal women. Although these details may seem unnecessary and a little confusing, understanding these differences will help you understand the rationale behind estrogen—and progesterone—replacement therapy.

Effects of Estrogen on Various Tissues

	Too Little	Too Much
Breasts	Atrophy (shrinks)	Tenderness, swelling
Vagina	Atrophy; dry and easily irritated	No real effect; may cause bleeding
Uterus	Atrophy; may have no periods or very light periods	Overgrowth of uterine lining, fibroids, heavy bleeding, endometrial cancer (Beware: Sometimes "absent" periods may be due to overgrowth and can result in hemorrhage and precancerous lesions.)
Skin	Drying and wrinkling	Bloating and fluid retention
Cardiovascular system	Possibly increased risk of heart attacks	Increased risk of strokes and heart attacks
Body fat	Midriff bulge; fat tends to collect around abdomen	Bloating, fluid retention; fat tends to occur on hips and thighs
Fertility	Anovulation (no eggs)	Anovulation
Hair	Thinning of hair on head	Head hair becomes thicker
Typical general complaints	Hot flashes, vaginal dryness, irritability, mood swings	Bloating, breast tenderness and fullness, nausea

In premenopausal women, the major estrogen is estradiol. After menopause, the estrogen estrone plays a larger role. Estrogenic hormones can be made in the ovaries, adrenal glands, and skin and fatty tissue. Prior to menopause, the major source of estrogen seems to be estradiol from the ovary. After menopause, the principal source of estrogen seems to be estrone made from peripheral (skin and fatty tissue) conversion of adrenal steroids such as androstenedione and testosterone. Seem confusing? It is, but if you keep in mind that your own hormonal balance results from a complex interaction between ovaries, adrenal glands, and fatty tissue and skin interconversion of steroid hormones, it is easier to understand how much individual variation in hormone levels there can be.

In premenopausal women, increasing preovulatory levels of estrogen enhance the pituitary response, which activates luteinizing hormone (LH) and brings about ovulation. Estrogen and progesterone support the processes that later produce the ovum and prepare the endometrium to receive the fertilized egg.

In perimenopausal women, ovulatory cycles are less frequent. After menopause, secretion of estrogen and progesterone by the ovaries stops almost completely. Then, peripheral conversion of androstenedione produces circulating estrogen.

In Chapter 1 we saw how estrogen and progesterone stimulate female pubertal changes, such as growth and maturation of the uterus, breasts and vaginal and urethral mucosa. When circulating levels of estrogen are reduced after menopause, these same target organs show effects—for example, cessation of menstruation, vaginal dryness, and urinary incontinence.

AN UPDATE ON ERT

Since synthetic estrogens first became available in the late 1940s, their popularity has followed a roller-coaster course. Oral estrogen therapy became enormously popular after Robert Wilson's best seller, *Feminine Forever* (New York: M. Evans and Company; Philadelphia, Penn.: J. B. Lippincott, 1966), hailed estrogens as a cure-all for wrinkling, sagging, and aging.

Then, in the early 1970s, hormones began to get some poor reviews.

Medical research reports appeared linking ERT with an increased risk of endometrial cancer (cancer of the lining of the uterus). Other reports appeared linking the use of DES (diethylstilbestrol, a synthetic estrogen) during pregnancy to the appearance of a rare but deadly vaginal cancer in daughters exposed to DES *in utero*.

At the same time, the rise of consumerism and the women's health movement and the end of the honeymoon for oral contraceptives combined to create a healthy public skepticism toward hormonal therapy in general. Sales of estrogens fell rapidly. Physicians quickly took many women off all hormones and refused to start estrogen replacement in other women.

Then, support for ERT emerged from several surprisingly divergent areas. First, many of the women taken off hormones complained bitterly: they suffered debilitating hot flashes and mood swings and believed that years of agony now were far worse than taking their chances of a possibly slightly increased risk of endometrial cancer 20 years hence.

Secondly, statisticians pointed out that while the incidence of endometrial cancer was increased, the cancers that occurred were almost without exception early and treatable, and that death rates were not increased by the use of estrogens.

Thirdly, gynecologists maintained that estrogens *were* safe for the large number of women who had had hysterectomies and were obviously immune to uterine cancers. Many physicians also believed that careful examination by uterine biopsies for precancerous changes allowed for safe use of ERT in women under careful medical surveillance.

Then, an unexpected entry into the controversy came from researchers in bone metabolism, who had long noted that some women who underwent premature menopause suffered a high rate of hip, wrist, and spinal compression fractures. Results of research began to appear that maintained that ERT could actually *reduce* the risk of such fractures, a major cause of hospitalization and death among elderly women. (See chapters 4 and 5.)

What initially looked like a hopeless dilemma—ERT both increased the risk of endometrial cancer and decreased the risk of bone fractures—seems to have had a happy resolution. Researchers observed that a hormone called progesterone reverses the effects of estrogen on the uterine lining without seeming to reverse its effects on bone. They believed that estrogen and progesterone given in combination might enhance bony strength without promoting endometrial cancer.

Epidemiologists also noted two significant findings:

- Women on birth control pills that were combinations of estrogen and progesterone had a lower risk of endometrial cancer than the general population.
- Women on the early formulations of birth control pills that had been high in estrogen and low in progesterone (the old "sequential" pills) had an increased risk of endometrial cancer.

Thus researchers determined that the increase in endometrial cancer perhaps was not caused by estrogen therapy itself, but rather by the fact that the doses used during the 1950s were too high and lacked progesterone balance to maintain normal endometrial growth.

Physicians experimented with a combination of estrogens and progestins that would mimic the normal menstrual cycle, believing that this would be the most natural and presumably safest way to use ERT.

The concept of adding cyclic progestogens to enhance endometrial shedding in estrogen-treated postmenopausal women was introduced in England in 1971. Early studies indicated that about 10 days of progestin therapy may only reverse 98% of endometrial overgrowth. R. Don Gambrell,

Jr., **M.D.**, Clinical Professor of Endocrinology and Obstetrics and Gynecology, Medical College of Georgia, Augusta, Georgia, writing in *The Female Patient* (July 1985), suggests that a more appropriate course of cyclic progestogens should be about 13 days each month. "This is because during the reproductive years, a woman's corpus luteum produces progesterone for 13 to 14 days during the normal 28-day ovulatory cycle. It seems logical for estrogen-treated women to take progestogens for at least the same number of days during a 30 or 31 day month," he says.

Dr. Gambrell outlined the concept of the Progestogen Challenge Test (PCT). He advises that all postmenopausal women with an intact uterus, regardless of symptoms, should have the PCT. A positive response, indicated by withdrawal bleeding, indicates that progestogen should be continued for 13 days each month as long as withdrawal bleeding follows. If there is no response, the PCT should be repeated each year.

Studies using the PCT and progestogens have reduced the incidence of endometrial cancer and breast cancer.

In the mid-1980s, most physicians prescribe estrogen by itself for 21 to 25 days out of the month, and add an oral progestin during at least the last 10 days of the estrogen. During the remaining days, women are off medication, allowing the lining of the uterus to shed and a light menstrual period to occur. Dosages of medications vary with the exact formulation and with the dose needed to eliminate hot flashes and other symptoms for each woman.

So far, results of combined estrogen-progestin therapy (E/PRT) are encouraging, with no evidence to date of increased risk of either uterine or breast cancer and considerable evidence that this combination may protect against osteoporosis and ultimately bone fractures.

However, women still have legitimate questions about the safety of long-term E/PRT. Many of the concerns researchers have regarding ERT relate to effects on breast tissue, on the uterus, on bones, on the cardiovascular system, and on the liver and gallbladder.

SOME UNANSWERED QUESTIONS ABOUT ERT

Effects on Breast Tissue

Breast tissue is stimulated by estrogens; certain breast cancers grow more rapidly when estrogens (either the body's own or synthetic) are present. Thus there is still concern about whether ERT increases a woman's risk of breast cancer.

Overall, while research data are inconclusive, a few studies claim an increased risk, but the bulk of studies show no effect. Because estrogens seem to *enhance* rather than *cause* the growth of breast cancers, a reasonable approach is to examine women carefully by breast examination and mammography for preexisting breast cancer but not to avoid ERT as long as exam and mammogram indicate that no breast cancer is present. Interestingly, several recent reports have indicated that E/PRT may actually *reduce* the risk of breast cancer in some women. However, it is too soon to know if this is a valid finding. Most physicians still avoid ERT in women who have a history of any previously estrogen-sensitive tumor.

Effect on the Uterus

A *New England Journal of Medicine* article reported an approximately sixfold increase in the risk of endometrial cancer in women on estrogen therapy for less than five years, and a 15-fold increase in long-term users (C. M. F. Antunes, P. D. Stolley, N. T. Rosenheim et al., "Endometrial Cancer and Estrogen Use: Report of a Large Case-Control Study," *New England Journal of Medicine* 300 [1979]: p. 9). A later article reported that the association between estrogen use and endometrial cancer may be overestimated because of a bias in detection (R. I. Horwitz and A. R. Reinstein, "Alternative Analytic Methods for Case-Control Studies of Estrogens and Endometrial Cancer," *New England Journal of Medicine* 299 [1978]: p. 1089). However, any risk could be reduced by appropriate attention to uterine bleeding and/or supplemental use of progestins.

Effect on the Bones

After reading chapters 4 and 5, you may see better how estrogen affects your bones. The *specific* role of estrogen is still unclear, even to researchers. However, it *is* known that bone mass visibly (on X ray or special bone density studies as described in chapters 4 and 5) deteriorates within one to two years of natural or artificial menopause. Estrogen seems to help prevent bone loss indirectly through interaction with another hormone called calcitonin.

Current research into the interactions of estrogen, parathyroid hormone, calcitonin, Vitamin D, calcium, phosphorus, fluoride, and the function of organs as diverse as the parathyroid glands in the neck and the kidneys may help sort out more specifically what happens in the bones when osteoporosis occurs.

Perhaps the time will come when a dietary suppplement containing the proper balance of calcium, fluoride, Vitamin D, and even calcitonin or parathyroid hormone may be used to prevent osteoporosis. Until that time, however, we are left with E/PRT as a somewhat indirect and not well explained preventive therapy.

Effect on the Cardiovascular System

High doses of estrogens are known to increase the risk of strokes and heart attacks. Doses currently in use of both E/PRT and oral contraceptives are considerably safer than the doses used during the 1960s. Still, there is concern that for some women, even currently used doses of both estrogens and progestins may increase the risk of cardiovascular disease. These risks are almost certain to be higher in women with other cardiovascular risk factors, such as smoking, obesity, high cholesterol or triglyceride levels (fatty substances in the blood), or personal or family history of heart disease.

In fall 1985, two studies in the *New England Journal of Medicine* (October 24, 1985) reported conflicting results regarding estrogens and cardiovascular disease. One said estrogen reduced, and the other said estrogen increased, the risk of heart disease. One analyzed data from the Framingham Heart Study, a collection of health statistics about residents of a Massachusetts town. Researchers followed up on 1,234 postmenopausal women who had been questioned between 1970 and 1972 about their use of estrogen. Of these women, 302 had used estrogens after menopause; 932 had not. Eight years later, the estrogen users had healthier scores than nonusers on risk factors known to be associated with cardiovascular disease including blood pressure, weight, and blood level of total cholesterol and its individual components. However, despite apparent advantages, the researchers reported that "significant detrimental effects were seen for total cardiovascular disease, coronary heart disease and stroke in particular." The researchers concluded that "no benefits from estrogen use were observed in the study group."

The other study in the same issue of the *New England Journal of Medicine* suggested that estrogens protect against heart disease. Six Harvard University researchers analyzed data collected in a long-term project in which periodic questionnaires were mailed to 121,964 female nurses who were between ages 30 and 55 in 1976. The Harvard researchers found that, overall, the death rate from heart disease among the nurses who had used estrogens was half that of the women who had never used them. They said duration of estrogen treatment was not a factor.

An editorial in the same issue of the *New England Journal of Medicine* said: "What are we to believe at this point? I simply cannot tell from present evidence whether these hormones add to the risk of various cardiovascular diseases, dimish the risk or leave it unchanged, and must resort to the investigator's great cop-out: More research is needed."

Another report in the same issue showed an increased risk of endometrial cancer not just in women currently using estrogens, but in past users as well.

More research may result in better information about dose levels and formulations that are safe for all women, but, currently, women with any risk factors should use E/PRT only with extreme caution and close supervision by a physician.

Effect on the Liver/Gallbladder

Pregnancy, oral contraceptive use, and use of E/PRT are all suspected as causes of certain types of gallbladder and liver problems. Gallstones are common in pregnant women and seem to be aggravated by high doses of estrogens. Oral contraceptives seem to cause benign liver tumors. Severe liver disease (fatty liver of pregnancy) is a rare, but often fatal, pregnancy complication. Therefore, women with known liver disease or gallbladder problems should be extremely cautious about E/PRT use.

If a woman with liver disease takes estrogens, she should know that because estrogens are metabolized (broken down) in the liver, she may not metabolize a standard dose and hence will have higher blood levels than would a woman with normal liver function. The dose for a woman with liver disease should be lower than for a comparable woman without liver disease.

Eventually, skin patches or vaginal creams may be able to deliver appropriate amounts of estrogen without the liver breakdown required for oral estrogens, perhaps making the skin patches more appropriate for women with liver disease.

AMA's GUIDELINES REGARDING ESTROGEN USE

The American Medical Association's Guidelines for use of estrogen in menopause, adopted in 1982 in an AMA Council on Scientific Affairs report, appeared in the January 21, 1983, issue of the *Journal of the American Medical Association*:

> *Estrogen replacement therapy has proved useful in controlling the "hot flashes" associated with the menopause and in relieving the irritation and painful intercourse that can result from atrophy of vaginal tissue. Estrogen therapy has been most effective in arresting or retarding loss of bone substance (osteoporosis) that increases the risk of fractures in postmenopausal women.*

Research analyzed for the report suggests that women treated with estrogen daily for two to four years have up to eight times the risk of developing uterine cancer as untreated women. The risk seems to decline after therapy is discontinued, however, and no increase in the death rate from uterine cancer has been noted, possibly because tumors in estrogen-treated women seem to be less "aggressive." In fact, the risk of death is less than that attributed to smoking one pack of cigarettes a day, the report says.

Other unwelcome side effects of estrogen replacement therapy include abnormal uterine bleeding, fluid retention, breast enlargement and growth of preexisting benign uterine tumors commonly called "fibroids."

As with any form of drug therapy, estrogens should be used only for responsive indications, in the smallest effective dose and for the shortest period that satisfies therapeutic need, the report recommends. In addition, physicians are warned to monitor the cumulative dosage of estrogen ointments and creams applied to vaginal tissues and to examine at least annually women treated with estrogen, even though they may not complain of symptoms.

Recent evidence also suggests that estrogen replacement may protect against atherosclerotic heart disease and heart attacks.

DETERMINE YOUR OWN RISK/BENEFIT PROFILE

> *"I'm too old to carry Kotex around all the time. I'm 59, take estrogen replacement, and have regular bleeding episodes that last 15 days each month. I've changed doctors twice. No one seems to regulate my dosage. Warn your readers about estrogen. It helps symptoms but creates more problems."*

> *"I intend to menstruate for as long as possible! The benefits with it (ERT) far outweigh the negatives."*

You should have a gynecologic examination once a year. Your doctor will evaluate your past medical history and your current symptoms and complaints. It is important that your doctor ascertain that your health history or physical condition will not make hormonal therapy unsafe for you.

Your complete physical examination should include a breast examination and a pelvic exam (an internal exam of the reproductive organs). Your doctor may recommend a mammogram (a diagnostic X ray procedure to examine the breasts). A sample of cells from your cervix (mouth of the uterus) or vagina and possibly from your endometrium (lining of the uterus) may be taken and studied under a microscope. Your blood pressure and a sample of your blood may be taken for cholesterol and diabetes testing.

You should have yearly examinations to determine changes in your blood pressure and blood chemistry as well as changes in your menopausal symptoms. Based on each yearly evaluation, your doctor may recommend taking another sample of cells for analysis.

Before you agree to begin ERT, you and your physician should thoroughly evaluate how the advantages and disadvantages of therapy relate to you personally. Your decision should be based on a combination of factors, including the severity of your current symptoms and your past medical history.

Possible Advantages of ERT

- May relieve hot flashes
- May relieve vaginal dryness
- May relieve vaginal discomfort during sexual intercourse
- May relieve urinary tract problems
- May help prevent or reduce severity of osteoporosis
- May or *may not* improve emotional mood swings and depression

Possible Disadvantages of ERT

Many women take estrogen and estrogen and progestin therapy without any side effects. Many other women do notice side effects. Following are some of the most reported:

- Recurrence of monthly bleeding (periods again!)
- Fluid retention (This may make some conditions worse, such as migraine, heart diseases kidney disease, or asthma)
- Swelling of the body; weight gain
- Breast tenderness or enlargement
- Abdominal cramping
- Irritability
- Effects on the uterus (Estrogen may cause benign fibroid tumors of the uterus to get larger)
- Nausea and vomiting

Most of these can be controlled or eliminated by reducing the dose.

More Serious Disadvantages that Can also Occur

- Endometrial or uterine cancer
- Other cancers, such as tumors of the breast, cervix, vagina, or liver
- High blood pressure
- Gallbladder disease and gallstones
- Abnormal blood clotting
- Jaundice; women with a past history of jaundice (yellowing of the skin and white parts of the eyes) may get jaundice again during estrogen use (If this occurs, stop taking estrogen and see your doctor.)

WHAT TO ASK IF ESTROGEN REPLACEMENT THERAPY IS RECOMMENDED FOR YOU

- Are my symptoms severe enough to warrant use of estrogen replacement therapy?
- Am I far enough along in my menopausal course to warrant taking estrogen replacement?
- Am I too far past menopause for estrogen therapy to do me much good?
- If my periods haven't stopped yet, will taking estrogen cause me to continue having periods past a reasonable menopausal age?
- What changes should I expect in my periods if I am still menstruating regularly? Heavier, lighter, spaced further apart?
- If I haven't menstruated in 10 years, will estrogen cause my periods to start again?
- How will estrogen affect my weight and the size of my breasts?
- How will I recognize symptoms that signal danger and that I should go off of hormone replacement? How will I know? How will my doctor know?

Should You Consider Beginning Estrogen/Progestin Therapy?

Here's what some of the respondents in the Holt-Kahn research asked/said:

> "I'd like a discussion in your book about the pros and cons of use of hormones. My doctor prescribed them for me but I refused to take them. I was a guinea pig for the birth control pill with disasterous results and am not comfortable with the idea."

> "I am bewildered and concerned about my symptoms. What do they really mean? Should I take hormones?"

> "E and P simply saved my life this year!"

> "Hormones have been extremely helpful. I am functioning as I did before menopause."

> "After hysterectomy, I had mood changes I did not realize were caused by hormone changes. I had a shaky 18 months till I adjusted with hormone therapy."

Who Should Consider Hormone Therapy?

- Women who undergo either surgical or natural menopause prior to age 50. Ovarian estrogens prior to menopause promote bone strength. The average age of menopause in the United States is 50, and women whose ovaries are removed or cease functioning at an earlier age are at particular risk of osteoporosis.

- Women with a family history of osteoporosis. As the disease does run in families, women whose female relatives had hip, wrist, or spinal fractures from relatively minor accidents should think about E/PRT.

- Women with a history of amenorrhea (no periods). Some women who have gone for long stretches without menstrual periods may have had low estrogen levels and be at high risk for osteoporosis. Underweight women, women with "stress amenorrhea," and athletes such as distance runners and gymnasts may be particularly prone to this problem.

- Smokers. Women who smoke, possibly due to a combination of poor diet and direct toxic effects of smoking on their bones, have higher osteoporosis rates. However, as smokers also are at increased risk for cardiovascular disease, physicians should be particularly careful about prescribing hormones for these women. Obviously, quitting cigarettes would be the most valuable approach for a smoker!

- Petite women. Taller women have larger bones; women under 5'2" often have more delicate bone structures.

- Caucasian and Oriental women. Black women have slightly denser, stronger bones and are less prone to osteoporosis.

- Women who have poor diets. A well-balanced diet adequate in calcium, zinc, phosphorus, fluoride, and vitamins is essential for good bone strength. (See chapter 8 to learn more about what a good diet for mature women includes.) Subgroups of women who often fall under the "poor diet" category include:
  - Alcoholic women or heavy drinkers. These women often have poor diets.
  - Women with many closely spaced pregnancies. Even if their diets have been adequate, few women can eat well enough to make up for the calcium demands of multiple pregnancies that occurred close together.

WHO SHOULD *NOT* CONSIDER TAKING ESTROGEN THERAPY

In general, women with the following health problems should avoid estrogen therapy:

- Women with a history of breast cancer
- Women with a history of endometrial (uterine) cancer

• Women with a history of cardiovascular disease
• Women with liver or gallbladder disease

(There may be exceptions to these guidelines. For example, for a woman with severe bone disease, the benefits might outweigh the risks. Also, a woman who is many years past breast cancer treatment might be considered a candidate for ERT. If you have any of these risk factors, however, be sure you have a physician who seems knowledgeable and attentive to your symptoms, not one who seems cavalier and unconcerned about possible complications.)

Hormonal therapy does *not* seem to *cause* breast cancer, but some cancers may grow more quickly under the "promoting" effects of E/PRT. Most physicians do not prescribe E/PRT for women with a history of breast cancer. Any woman at all concerned about breast disease should insist on a thorough breast exam and a mammogram before initiating E/PRT.

In light of recent evidence that estrogens and progestins combined may actually *protect* against breast cancer, however, some physicians are starting to use E/PRT in carefully selected former cancer patients who seem to be totally free of cancer, particularly if studies at the time their cancer was diagnosed indicate that the tumor was not sensitive to hormonal stimulation.

The same line of reasoning as to breast cancer applies to women who have had endometrial cancer.

Although the currently used doses of estrogens and progestins are less risky than the high doses used in early ERT and oral contraceptives, it is still uncertain whether current doses are safe for women with heart disease (severe high blood pressure, stroke, pulmonary embolus, heart attack, or other major heart conditions).

For some women, the benefits of E/PRT might outweigh the risks, but such women and their doctors should use E/PRT cautiously, at as low a dose as possible, and with careful attention to possible cardiovascular side effects such as chest pain, worsening migraine headaches, or blood clots.

Benign liver tumors also have been associated with the use of oral contraceptives. Women who use estrogens after menopause are more likely to develop gallbladder disorders needing surgery than women who do not use estrogens. Since estrogens are metabolized (broken down) in the liver, women with impaired liver function may require lower doses than women who have normal liver function. Again, for each woman, the benefits of E/PRT may outweigh the risks, but extreme caution should be used, especially by women who have liver or gallbladder disease.

Physicians recommend that women who had blood clotting in the legs or lungs or a heart attack or stroke while using birth control pills should not use estrogen for menopausal symptoms, except in very individual and carefully supervised circumstances.

MORE Words of Warning About
Estrogen Replacement Therapy

If you decide to take estrogens, you can do so as safely as possible by understanding that your doctor will want you to have regular physical examinations while you are taking them, will try to discontinue the drug as soon as possible, and will use the smallest dose possible. After you start taking them, be alert for signs of trouble, including:

- Abnormal vaginal bleeding (you can expect a light flow on your "off" days)
- Pains in your calves, or chest, or sudden shortness of breath, or coughing blood
- Severe headache, dizziness, faintness, or changes in vision
- Breast lumps
- Jaundice (yellowing of the skin)
- Severe depression not attributable to other factors

Remember, your prescription for estrogen replacement therapy was designed individually for you. Do not share your prescription with a friend. Her needs will be different from yours. Do not give your estrogen medication, or any other medication prescribed for you, to anyone else.

Summing Up Your Personal Benefit/Risk Profile

"My menopause was so simple. I believe a woman's state of mind can lessen the need for pills or hormones. Acceptance of herself as a complete person with or without the ability to bear children is so important to the menopausal transition."

"Take hormones with menopause if problems exist and your doctor recommends it. Do not suffer unnecessarily."

In view of such unexpected tragedies as vaginal cancers in women exposed *in utero* to DES, both the medical community and the average woman are wary of possible unsuspected risks later on from hormone replacement now. Could there be long-term complications that we have not even suspected? This fear of the unknown is legitimate, but should be balanced against what for some women are severe side effects of untreated menopause, such as debilitating hot flashes, chronic vaginal discomfort, and the chance of osteoporosis.

Some risks are known; others are not. Benefits and risks vary from woman to woman. Using the information in this chapter and throughout this book, you can develop your own benefit/risk profile and make an informed decision.

"I'd like the straight 'scoop' on whether hormone additives are safe and will they help retard the aging processes. Basically, I don't like interfering with the body's natural processes."

HOW IS ESTROGEN TAKEN?

If your doctor advises ERT for you, your prescription will call for the type that will affect target tissues with minimum side effects. The goal of therapy is to relieve specific symptoms with the lowest effective dose.

The effect on the body of the synthetic estrogens and progestins is similar to but not exactly the same as that of the natural compounds. The strength and possible side effects differ depending on the chemical structure and route of administration. Most physicians say they prescribe a dose of conjugated estrogen 0.3 to 1.25 milligrams, or the equivalent, daily and cyclically. When symptoms such as hot flashes cease, doses are often reduced gradually and eventually the therapy is discontinued.

Conjugated estrogens are biologically produced estrogens (often from horse urine) that contain several forms of estrogens similar to the varied forms naturally found in the human body. These are most widely used for ERT in the United States. Synthetic forms of estrogen (mestranol, ethinyl estradiol) are a single form of estrogen. These are more potent hormones; at present it is unclear whether conjugated or synthetic estrogens are preferable. In some instances one might be better tolerated; side effects may occur with one form and not another although most side effects are dose related.

Estrogens and progestins currently are available for use in four forms:

- Orally
- By injection
- Topically (outside the body)
- As a patch worn on the skin

In the future, similar medications may be available for use:

- As an implant under the skin

Oral Tablets

In the United States, the most popular form of estrogen therapy is in tablets taken orally. Usual therapy is 0.625 milligrams of conjugated estrogens daily for the first three weeks of every four (as with oral contraceptives) or the first 25 days of each calendar month

Advantages

- Easy to take, can be stopped, can be taken intermittently
- A progestin can be added daily for the last 7 to 14 days of each cycle to avoid overstimulation of the endometrium

Disadvantages

- Monthly bleeding sometimes results
- There frequently is a peak and valley curve of drug levels in the blood (At times, the drug concentration is too high, causing side effects; or too low, becoming ineffective.)

Injected Estrogen

Advantage

- Trouble-free most of the month; patient does not have to remember daily schedule

Disadvantages

- Requires a visit to the doctor
- Not appropriate for long-term use
- Androgens, occasionally combined with the injection, may cause problems of hirsutism and voice changes
- Difficult to cycle with progestins because of dose
- Difficult to control level of hormone—may initially be too high, later too low

Vaginal Estrogens (Topical)

In the Holt-Kahn survey, only 2.9% of the nonphysician respondents reported using estrogen creme vaginally; however, 3.8% of the women gynecologists use it.

Advantages

- Estrogen is well-absorbed through the vaginal walls and enters the circulation for distribution

- Delivers a good dose to vaginal area when a major indication is vaginal dryness
- Can produce blood levels close to those attained with oral estrogen
- Useful for patients who comply with therapeutic regimen when they perceive local effects

"When I told my doctor about my problem of discomfort during intercourse because of vaginal dryness, he prescribed vaginal estrogen creme. I misundertood how I was to use it and used it as a lubricant with my husband. It works." [Occasionally, however, a male partner could absorb enough estrogen to have side effects.]

Disadvantages

- Absorption is uncontrolled; estrogen circulates through the body before reaching the liver.
- Dose may be excessive since large variation may occur in dose absorbed.
- Hormones have systemic effects (effects throughout the body) even though the woman may believe she is being treated externally.

Transdermal Patch

The transdermal patch may improve the therapeutic regimen of hormone substitution by improving the balance of beneficial versus adverse effects. Transdermal therapy works by placing a patch, containing medication, or in this case, hormones, on the woman's skin. The medication is delivered directly through the skin and into the bloodstream.

Advantages

- This route circumvents the first pass through the liver, decreasing the possibility of liver damage
- Medication goes through the skin and into the bloodstream, so that a lower dose is needed
- Gradual, constant delivery may reduce or eliminate the side effects of some estrogen medications
- May eliminate hot flashes with a lower dose of medication
- Drugs remain in the therapeutic range throughout the life of the patch
- Patches are easy to administer, to wear, and to remove

Disadvantages

- Some transdermal medications may cause allergic reactions of the skin
- It is unclear whether skin patches will offer protection against osteoporosis
- As with any new product, it may be years before all possible problems are appreciated.

In the future, similar medications may be available in an additional way:

Subcutaneous Implantation

Advantages

- Convenient if duration of therapy is long
- Small, continuously released dose avoids the peak/valley problem of oral administration

Disadvantages

- Continuous stimulation of the endometrium
- Little control of absorption
- Exposure to hormone can't be easily interrupted
- Probably will require insertion and removal by a medical professional

Determining the dosage

How do you—or your doctor—know if you are taking enough estrogen? Or too much? From the viewpoint of preventing osteoporosis, the optimal dose seems to be 0.625 milligrams of conjugated estrogens, 1 milligram of 17ß-estradiol, or 15 micrograms of ethinyl estradiol (approximately half of the dose in low-dose, 35-microgram oral contraceptives).

To help prevent uterine cancer, most authorities recommend using for at least 10 days out of the month a dose of 5 milligrams of norethindrone acetate or 10 milligrams of medroxyprogesterone acetate.

Remember, these doses may have to be adjusted downward to prevent side effects, and more estrogen may be needed to prevent hot flashes for an individual woman. Doses may be adjusted downward if you have any of the following side effects:

- Nausea
- Breast swelling
- Fluid retention
- Bloating
- Acne
- Irritability from the progestin
- Unwelcome "periods" on the off-days

Many women are unhappily surprised to find out that they have "periods" on the off-days (unless, of course, they have had hysterectomies), and most gynecologists are pleased if their patients have light flow *only* during the off-days. Midcycle bleeding (bleeding during the medication) must be investigated, often by a sampling of the uterine lining and a Pap smear to be sure no precancerous or cancerous condition exists. Most midcycle bleeding is not dangerous and usually can be eliminated after a thorough investigation by slight adjustments in the amounts or durations of either estrogen or progesterone.

MYTH VS. TRUTH?

Better skin, sex, sense of well-being? There is actually little scientific evidence that ERT has any direct effect on skin tone, sex life, or mood swings.
However:
Skin: Many women insist that their skin seems more elastic and less dry (i.e., younger looking) with ERT. But, heredity, a good diet, and avoidance of cigarette smoke and sun are probably more important in maintaining a healthy skin. And it is questionable whether we should consider "young-looking" skin our primary goal. But for what it's worth, this is an area many women claim as a benefit of ERT.
Sex life: Similarly, ERT is not proven to affect libido. However, since it can solve vaginal dryness and painful intercourse, needless to say many women are more interested in sex after taking ERT. Many women insist as well that their libido improves on ERT, although again there is little scientific support for this assertion.
Sense of well-being: Many women insist that ERT cures the mood swings so many women identify with menopause. We would not argue with success for the women who feel this way, but would mainly caution that women with severe depression should seek professional help.

ROLE OF ESTROGEN IN PROTECTING WOMEN AGAINST CARDIOVASCULAR DISEASE

Use of estrogen replacement therapy in protecting women against atherosclerotic cardiovascular disease is somewhat controversial, as described earlier in this chapter.

Up until menopausal age, women seem to have fewer cardiovascular problems than men. After age 50, the incidence of heart disease among women goes up, and around age 70, the chances of either sex developing heart disease are about the same.

Some researchers believed that estrogen protected younger women. Now they aren't so sure. Several studies in which relatively high doses of estrogen were given to men who had previously had acute heart attack, or who were being treated for cancer of the prostate, showed an increase in the rate of atherosclerotic disease and acute myocardial infarction.

It may be that older women develop heart problems at a higher rate than younger women simply because of age and also because of levels of fat in the blood. Additional estrogen may not prevent these changes. However, in women who have had a premature menopause, estrogen therapy may help prevent premature heart disease. Recent evidence suggests that low-dose progesterone may be the protective agent for women prior to menopause.

NONHORMONAL MEDICATIONS USED DURING AND AFTER MENOPAUSE

According to the American College of Obstetricians and Gynecologists, if estrogen replacement therapy is contraindicated for a woman who has severe menopausal symptoms, other medications may be helpful.

To reduce the incidence of hot flashes, medroxyprogesterone acetate and D-norgestrel have been effective for some women. Some sedatives and psychopharmacologic agents may also reduce hot flashes, but studies are not yet conclusive.

To prevent osteoporosis, many approaches have been recommended, such as drinking milk, exercising, and taking calcium supplements, calcitonin, Vitamin D, and fluorides (see chapters on osteoporosis).

The American College of Obstetricians and Gynecologists says that there is no good alternative therapy for vaginal atrophy, but adds that painful intercourse may be partially relieved by the use of lubricants (see chapter 2).

According to Wulf H. Utian, M.D., in *Menopause in Modern Perspective* (New York: Appleton-Century-Crofts, 1980), nonhormonal drugs have a secondary role in the management of menopausal symptoms. He suggests four groups of women for whom nonhormonal drugs may be recommended:

- Those for whom hormonal therapy is contraindicated
- Those who do not respond to sex-steroid therapy
- Those who do not want hormone therapy but want symptom relief
- Those who cannot tolerate sex-steroids because of side effects such as nausea or fluid retention

Nonhormonal treatments include sedatives, tranquilizers, antidepressants, and drugs such as clonidine and propranolol, vitamins, and even therapies prescribed by practitioners of Oriental medicine.

Tranquilizers

Tranquilizers comprise a large group of drugs that may be overprescribed, especially for mature women whose complaints strike many physicians as vague and nonspecific. However, for some women, tranquilizers may be helpful adjuncts to psychotherapeutic programs, especially if the woman is excessively anxious, agitated, irritable, or insomniac.

Tranquilizers are often prescribed for short durations during periods of explainable stress, such as during divorce proceedings, or immediately after the death of a husband or other loved one. If you take tranquilizers during such times, wean yourself off of them gradually, as soon as possible. Instead, substitute exercise and new interests.

The most frequently prescribed tranquilizers include:
Diazepam
Chlordiazepoxide
Benzodiazepine
Hydroxyzine
Meprobamate
Phenothiazines
Barbiturates

All are available under different brand names.

Avoid physicians who seem to "push" sedatives and tranquilizers without completely evaluating your symptoms and lifestyle.

Antidepressants

Mood changes due to normal life stresses around the time of menopause and after usually are not enough to warrant taking antidepressant drugs. This class of drugs should be reserved for true psychiatric depression.

The most frequently prescribed antidepressants include:
Amitriptyline
Monoamine-oxidase (MAO) inhibitors
Dibenzoxepin tricyclic compounds
Imipramines
Lithium

Recent advances in our understanding of the chemical imbalances involved in depression (which runs in families), and more sophisticated antidepressants, have led to wider use of these agents. Some people are trying them for PMS sufferers and victims of Alzheimer's disease; they are being used with success in certain patients who have chronic pain.

Certainly, antidepressants should be used only when necessary; and as with tranquilizers, you should sense that your doctor is looking at the big picture and suggesting such medication in combination with, not instead of, treating your "whole self."

Since antidepressants can have serious side efects, become very familiar with potential risks as well as with interactions with other medications and foods, if any drugs in the antidepressant category are prescribed for you. Antidepressants also interreact with other medications. Be wary.

Clonidine

Clonidine is a derivative of imidazoline, which some researchers during the 1970s believed reduced the severity and frequency of hot flashes. It is also used as an antihypertensive and as an antimigraine drug. Further research is needed to determine whether clonidine may be effective for reducing severe menopausal symptoms in women who cannot take ERT (J. R. Clayden, "Effect of Clonidine on Menopausal Flushing," *Lancet* 2 [1972]: p. 1361; J. R. Clayden, J. W. Bell, and P. Pillard, "Menopausal Flushing—Double Blind Trial of a Non-Hormonal Medication," *British Medical Journal* 1 [1974]: p. 409; R. Lindsay and D. M. Hart, "Failure of Response of Menopausal Vasomotor Symptoms to Clonidine," *Maturitas* 1 [1978]: p. 21).

Studies have shown that clonidine may reduce cravings during withdrawal from cigarettes, alcohol, and opiates. This may occur because clonidine controls the ability of the brain to produce too much noradrenalin, a chemical that contributes to the irritability and anxiety that goes along with withdrawal.

Propranolol

Propranolol is currently the most popular of a class of drugs known as beta-blockers, which inhibit the blood vessel-constricting effects of adrenalin-like hormones in the body. Propranolol is effective in relieving some heart symptoms and migraine headaches. However, studies have not shown that it is effective in relieving menopausal hot flashes (J. Coope, S. Williams, and J. S. Patterson, "A Study of the Effectiveness of Propranolol in Menopausal Hot Flashes," *British Journal of Obstetrics and Gynecology* 85 [1978]: p. 472).

Vitamin B₆ (Pyridoxine)

Researchers have found that certain estrogens and possibly progestogens lead to a deficiency of vitamin B_6 (pyridoxine). Deficiency of B_6 may bring about depression, fatigue, disturbances in concentration, mood swings, and possibly lack of interest in sexual activity. Some physicians give women on estrogens supplements of Vitamin B_6 (P. W. Adams, D. P. Rose, J. Folkart et al., "Effect of Vitamin B_6 upon Depression Associated with Oral Contraception," *Lancet* 1 [1973]: p. 897; A. A. Haspels, H. F. T. Coelingh, and W. H. P. Schreurs, "Disturbance of Tryptophan Metabolism and Its Correction During Estrogen Treatment in Postmenopausal Women," *Maturitas* 1 [1978]: p. 15).

ALTERNATIVE THERAPIES

Some women who have consulted physicians and not been satisfied with relief of symptoms may wish to try Oriental medicine, which may use herbal therapy and/or acupuncture or acupressure treatments.

Most American physicians will frown at you if you even suggest interest in these therapies. The authors neither endorse nor condemn them, but in a spirit of sharing, want you to know what we found during our research. However, if you choose to go this route, we sincerely hope that you have been thoroughly evaluated by reputable medical doctors to rule out cancer and other serious problems.

Practitioners of Oriental medicine say they take a "holistic" approach and look at the total of your body and mind rather than treating specific symptoms. They say that a healthy person is one who can use her or his full range of emotions in appropriate response to stimuli.

Their philosophy is "moderation in all things," according to William Dunbar, D.N., C.A., Director, Midwest Center for the Study of Oriental Medicine, Chicago. "A little sugar, fat, and cholesterol are allright. So is a little liquor. If there is an extreme craving for liquor, or for hot or cold foods, that may be a clue that something in your system is out of balance," he explains.

"Sleep and exercise are necessary, but not too much of either. Sex is necessary; too much or too little can damage your energy," he adds.

Oriental medicine teaches its adherents to be attuned to their own bodies. "Most of us are somewhat out of synchronization with nature. In winter, the ground rests. In spring, everything blossoms again. We should follow what the seasons show us," says Dr. Dunbar.

"Our ancestors laid low in winter, stayed indoors, repaired their tools, kept warm and slept a lot. We don't give our bodies a rest. That's why people are run down at the end of winter. Depression comes from using up too much energy. Emotions go with the physical energy, too," he says.

Regarding use of estrogen, Dr. Dunbar has this to say: "Taking estrogen may confuse your body's natural system and may cause what natural production is left to slow down." A woman should consult her prescribing physician, however, before changing or altering the dosage of any medication.

"Use of estrogen for menopausal symptoms may or may not be appropriate for all women because of individual differences," he explains. Chinese medicine is based on differential diagnosis (just as is Western medicine). Individual problems are diagnosed and treatments are individualized. Chinese remedies for hot flashes might differ for various menopausal women," he explains.

According to Dr. Dunbar, in Oriental medicine, diagnosis includes pulse taking and tongue examination. Pulses are taken at six different positions on each wrist; each position is thought to correspond to a body organ and its energy condition. The tongue is examined for size, color, coating, and moisture. (Not so different from the "stick out your tongue and say aaahhh" routine, is it?) These factors are said to give the diagnostician information about various pathways of energy and organs.

Says Dr. Dunbar, "A woman who has hot flashes probably has had some other disorders before she is menopausal. She may have had problems with menstruation, digestion, or stress. As a result of energy not moving properly through her body, she might have had PMS or menstrual irregularities. Around the time of menopause, hot flashes, vaginal infections and vaginal dryness might occur. She may have had an energetic imbalance for some time and we would treat that imbalance."

What Remedies?

For hot flashes, Oriental herbalists might formulate an herbal tea on an individual basis for each woman. It may take 8 to 10 different herbs, some of which have synergistic actions. Typical herbs are licorice, ginseng, coptis, and the Chinese form of rhubarb. Most of the herbs used by Oriental herbalists in the United States come from China.

Herbal medicine and acupuncture are not new. "They have been used by millions of people for thousands of years. More than two thirds of the world's population have received acupuncture during their lifetime.

Acupuncture was largely unknown until the opening of China to the Western world in 1972," explains Dr. Dunbar.

Chinese hospitals have extensive herb departments, stocked with remedies that have stood the test of time. Herbal remedies generally are not encouraged by American physicians because very few American clinical trials have been performed with them to scientifically prove their efficacy and/ or safety.

If you are considering herbal therapy, there are advantages and disadvantages, according to Julie Duffy, Ac.T., President, Illinois State Acupuncturists Association and Dean of Students at the Midwest Center for the Study of Oriental Medicine. Here they are:

Advantages

- No side effects
- Herbs don't mask symptoms, enabling therapist to treat the root cause to relieve the problem
- No known or anticipated long-range deleterious effects on the body

Disadvantages

- May be bad tasting
- Inconvenient to prepare; patient must cook herbs, boil, and strain them before drinking
- Available only in large metropolitan areas with large Asian communities
- Women might delay seeking appropriate medical attention for treatable conditions

Acupuncturists also treat hot flashes and menstrual irregularities by using specially designed needles at certain meridians, or lines on the body.

If you decide to consult an acupuncturist or specialist in Oriental medicine for any health problem, how can you determine if you are going to a reputable one? There are practitioners out there who have taken only 100 hours of instruction and are not board certified or licensed by any regulating body. Avoid those people.

In California, acupuncturists are licensed as primary care practitioners. In some other states, acupuncturists must also be licensed to practice. Whether or not licensure is required in your state, here are four questions to ask:

- Is the acupuncturist certified by the National Commission for the Certification of Acupuncture? (Call Manhasset, New York, (516) 627-0309 to ask.)

- Is the acupuncturist licensed in the state in which he or she practices? (Remember that not all states have acupuncture licenses.)
- Does the practitioner carry malpractice insurance?
- Is the practitioner a member of the state acupuncturists association (assuming there is one)?

According to the National Commission for the Certification of Acupuncture, at this time, there are more than 1,000 certified acupuncturists in the United States.

Remember that acupuncturists cannot prescribe drugs or perform surgery. However, acupuncture is performed by some M.D.s who have had special training; they can of course also prescribe ethical drugs and do surgery.

Most acupuncture practitioners are not M.D.s, but, in fact, have greater training in this speciality than M.D.s who practice acupuncture. "In many states, acupuncturists work hand in hand with medical doctors and we believe that acupuncture is *complementary* to Western medicine and not just an alternative," says Dr. Dunbar.

In some states, health insurance covers acupuncture treatments, depending on specific legislation in that state. California (at this time) is the only state that has a law requiring third party reimbursement for acupuncture therapy. However, many insurance companies will reimburse for treatment; you should file a claim.

If you would like more information about acupuncture or direction regarding acupuncture in your area, you may contact:

Midwest Center for the Study of Oriental Medicine
1222 West Grace Street
Chicago, Illinois 60613

"Westernized" Herbal Therapies

Herbs used by American herbal therapists are completely different from those used in Oriental medicine. American herbalists use herbs available in this country. For example, a feminist handbook prepared by the Feminist Health Works, New York, suggests an herbal remedy for hot flashes, dizziness, weakness, and emotional imbalance: "In some cases, red raspberry leaf tea alone has calmed nerves and eliminated hot flashes. It is a superior uterine tonic which contains progesterone- and estrogen-like substances, and vitamins to feed the adrenal and other glands. Those for whom raspberry is not adequate, should take other herbs in tincture or capsules on a daily basis to tone and regulate the endocrine and hormonal system."

Making their hot flash capsules requires powdering four different herbs in a blender and filling the capsules with the mixture. Their menopause tincture includes alfalfa, angelica, blessed thistle, comfrey, red raspberry leaves, sarsaparilla, saw palmetto berries, Siberian ginseng, and squaw vine, powdered, and mixed with cider vinegar or 100-proof vodka.

If you want more details, write to:

Feminist Health Works
487-A Hudson Street
New York, New York 10014

For additional information about herbal therapies, look at the book *Hygieia*, by Jeannine Parvati, published by Freestone Publishing Co., Berkeley, California 1983.

Other Specialists

Remember that many medical specialists take an interest in problems related to women's midlife health. Please see chapter 3 for brief descriptions of some medical specialties that you may also wish to consult.

WHAT'S THE FUTURE OF ESTROGEN REPLACEMENT THERAPY AND OTHER TREATMENTS FOR MENOPAUSAL SYMPTOMS?

Before our daughters are menopausal, we hope that researchers will make advancements in estrogen preparations that will result in more of the desired effects than currently used treatments, without so many side effects. Ideally, we hope to have a form of estrogen that would not stimulate growth of the lining of the uterus, but would have restorative effects on the vaginal wall, the urethra, and the bladder. It would not cause blood pressure to rise or body weight to increase. It would, however, have a calcium-retaining effect as well as an ability to ward off osteoporosis.

Also, we hope that routes of drug administration may be developed so that estrogens are not taken orally, with injection, or by implantation. We look foward to a new method of administration that would maintain beneficial blood plasma levels while reducing the number of side effects.

In the future, researchers may develop screening methods to determine which women might be at greatest risk for severe side effects or complications from estrogen therapy. This would enable more women to safely use estrogen replacement therapy without concern about the possible cancer-causing factors that worry our generation.

Additionally, use of other nonhormonal drugs to treat symptoms of menopause may be developed that would be helpful to the many women who cannot or are not willing to use estrogen replacement therapy in its current form.

7

BE ACTIVE!
KEEP YOUR MOVABLE
PARTS MOVING

"I found swimming the best kind of therapy during the menopausal years. I enrolled in classes at the YWCA, beginner's through advanced, and swam regularly. I'm 59 and still do."

"Be sure to stress the importance of good nutrition and exercise all through life, not just in midlife."

The best teachers about fitness are older women who have stayed agile. In this chapter, you'll read about how many midlife women—and one 79-year-old—keep themselves fit and help others do so, too. You'll find details on some women's attitudes about exercise, why good health depends on movement, what physical fitness means, the benefits of many popular forms of exercise, and some tips on fashion and safety during exercise.

There was a time when "horses sweat, men perspired, and women glowed." Not so anymore. Many midlife women today are out there sweating on jogging trails, on racketball courts, and in health clubs.

Despite all the visible women bending and stretching in colorful leotards, active sports and competition aren't for *all* midlife women. Many are mainly interested in keeping their bodies flexible and their movable parts moving as well as possible. Many want to build up their energy levels to the fullest capacity.

In the Holt-Kahn survey, 55.6% of respondents exercise regularly; 42.1% reported they do not (2.3% did not answer this question). Here's what some of the women said about exercise:

"If you exercise regularly, you'll whiz right through menopause."

"Food supplements and exercise are very important. Both have made me feel much better during this period."

"In response to your question about exercise, I'd like you to know that I have had barely enough strength to do my teaching and basic housework. I am feeling stronger now, nine months after my hysterectomy. I plan to begin aerobic dancing in an over-50 class."

YOUR BODY IS MEANT TO MOVE

"A round back is a picture of age. With a little effort, you can keep the picture of youth," says Anne Rudolph, a 79-year-old Chicagoan with flowing white hair who has researched and taught "self-applied body education" for more than half a century.

"When I was young, I asked students in their forties to do things. They said, 'Wait until you are our age!' You can't stop aging. But you can live the full length of your life with quality. I've never been this old before. But I can still leap into the air," (and she does, with agility and grace).

"Your body is meant to move. It needs motion to survive. Constant neglect of movement causes the body to signal its resentment with pain," she says. "That's why movement should be a lifelong study, yet we pay more attention to headaches than flexibility," she says.

Anne Rudolph has worked with people from every walk of life, from infants to 80-year-olds. Her students have been thousands of previously sedentary people, office workers, athletes, and amateur and professional dancers. Her work has been recognized and supported by medical and health authorities around the world. Her classes and philosophy appeal to many who consider themselves "unathletic" or "nondancers" but who are interested in improving and maintaining their flexibility.

"Hands have a purpose," she says, as she holds a small pillow in her hands. She flings the pillow on the floor in the middle of the room. She rises gracefully from the sofa, strides toward the pillow, bends, and reaches out with the full length of both arms to pick up the pillow. She tosses it into the air and catches it. "Full use of my limbs and muscles, that takes care of osteoporosis."

"The human body is an amazing piece of equipment. The spine is the most mind-boggling engineering feat known to man. Think of your body as a total unit, in which each part influences the other parts. Your body is a naturally aligned form designed to move and function harmoniously. It is capable of great resilience and strength."

"The trained body doesn't slouch or wobble. It moves as a single unit," says Anne. She considers walking upright "the most difficult thing man has ever done. Now we have to lift everything over two legs and two feet. No wonder we tilt back and forth, and have round shoulders and curvatures!"

Her message to tall women: "Don't slouch. Let others look up."

What's good exercise for midlife women? Women today don't find time for movement. Many of us have become merely "joint movers" instead of moving with our muscles. Without advocating any particular form of exercise beyond "controlled body movement," Anne emphasizes that midlife women can improve their flexibility.

To improve flexiblity at midlife, Anne advises thinking of yourself as a "mover through space" and concentrating on using basic muscle control in doing simple tasks, such as walking, reaching, or bending. She advocates using one's strength and muscle development as a way of achieving a better sense of well-being: "When a woman discovers the wonder of self-applied movement, she sheds her years and becomes more graceful and confident."

How much room do you need for a workout? "Stretch your arms out to the side and rotate them in large circles. That's all the space you need. When did you last have your arms stretched upward, over your head? Reach, stretch. Get your chest out. Lift your chin."

"The belly wall is the most difficult to keep under control at any age, and particularly at midlife. There are no bones to hold it up. It needs the support and power of bone and elasticity and springiness of muscle for help." What she teaches is to straighten your spine, pull back your shoulders, contract the muscles of your butt, and the muscles of your belly will go flat. It takes a lot of effort, but it works!

Anne's quick analysis of body problems comes from years of studying movement. At age 16, she was a top athlete, and at age 19, she made her dancing debut in Cologne, Germany, in Shakespeare's *As You Like It*. She considered training for the Olympics in broad jump, or running. She studied the "art of running" and determined that what really counted (in a 75-meter race) was *how* you got started. "After you start, there's no time to plan."

Anne headed her own school of body movement education in Germany, came to Chicago in 1934 on a three-month visit to learn about progressive athletics in the United States, met her husband-to-be, stayed in the United States, and soon opened her own school of body movement.

Anne is still an outstanding athlete; until recent years, she was jogging two miles a day with ease. "Now I think walking briskly is just right for me. When I walk, I think rhythm. I think, 1–2. I don't stop and take my pulse as I see so many people doing. While I walk, I hum, and that tells me if I'm getting out of breath. The first deep breath I take after I stop tells me how fast I'm back to normal."

Anne says, "Not everyone can be like me. But I hope more women will become more graceful, healthy individuals who can move powerfully and elegantly. I'd like more people to understand the concept of the beauty of a balanced body."

WHAT PHYSICAL FITNESS MEANS

"The average sedentary woman is subject to a loss of some physiological function after age 35," says Everett L. Smith, Ph.D., director of the Biogerontology Laboratory in the department of Preventive Medicine at the University of Wisconsin, Madison. "This loss can imperil her quality of life, when muscles weaken, decreased work capacity, stiffness and fractures make them unequal to the tasks of daily living. Much of this loss can be prevented or reversed through programs of physical activity. Women who start and stick to an exercise program at any age can look forward to a healthier and possibly better quality of life."

In addition to helping you feel better, physical activity plays a major role in bone maintenance, regardless of age, says Dr. Smith. In several studies, middle-aged women (35 to 64 years old) who exercised at least one hour a day, three days each week, showed greater arm density than sedentary women of the same age.

Keeping your bones strong is important enough, but being physically fit also means that you have enough energy for your daily routine of work and/or family life and still enough pep to enjoy recreational and social activities. Being physically fit means that you sleep well most of the time and get up each morning with enthusiasm for the day.

Physical fitness won't *make* you healthier or live longer. Health and fitness are not synonymous, although they certainly are related. Health is the absence of disease or injury; a fit body is a conditioned one.

Physical fitness can help you appear more attractive and confident, have better skin, maintain your weight so that your clothes fit for more than one season, cope with hot flashes (if you have them), decrease the threat of osteoporosis as you age, and increase your ability to live life to the fullest.

Additionally, you can derive specific benefits from regular exercise, as outlined by the President's Council on Physical Fitness:

- Increase your strength, endurance, and coordination
- Increase joint flexibility
- Reduce minor aches, pains, stiffness, and soreness
- Correct remediable postural defects
- Improve your general appearance
- Increase your efficiency with reduced expenditure of energy in performing both physical and mental tasks
- Improve your ability to relax and to voluntarily reduce tension
- Reduce chronic fatigue

Your individual level of physical fitness depends considerably on your personal combination of appropriate nutrition; adequate sleep and relaxation; good health habits, such as not smoking, and control of your intake of caffeine and alcohol; as well as your pattern of regular physical activity.

Because of today's conveniences, many midlife women are not as energetic during the activities of daily living as women of previous generations. "I carried 25 pails of coal into the house each day before we had radiator heat when I was a young girl," says Anne Rudolph, the 79-year-old proponent of "self-applied body movement." Hanging clothes out on a line gave many of our grandmothers good stretching and bending exercise. Working on farms gave women more exercise than we get sitting at computer terminals and taking elevators. Regular physical activity today is largely purposely planned. Many of us sign up for aerobic dance classes or schedule early morning half hours to jog, using the same motions that we avoid by using labor saving devices.

WHAT KIND OF EXERCISE IS FOR YOU?

It is always wise to consult your doctor before starting an exercise program. If you haven't been an exerciser, and you wonder what to do to improve your overall level of fitness, you aren't alone. Reinforcing this idea is Phyllis Perlman, R.N., nurse-psychotherapist, Bayshore, New York, who has counseled hundreds of women and men about physical fitness, exercise, weight control, and nutrition. "Many average hard-working couples who require two incomes just aren't sure what they should be doing for fitness. They need counseling. I've found that the level of physical fitness at midlife among some population groups needs improvement. Many are in poor physical shape."

Many need specially tailored exercise programs to meet individual needs. "I wouldn't suggest morning jogging for everyone." Perlman's recommendations for many of her clients include walking briskly for 20 to 30 minutes a day, four or five times a week; using the stationary bicycle for the same time periods; riding a bicycle outdoors; working out at gyms or health clubs; swimming two or three times a week; or dancing.

Hal Higdon, a world-class long-distance runner over age 50 and author of *Fitness After Forty* (Mountain View, Calif.: World Publications, 1977) said in a recent issue of *The Physician and Sportsmedicine*:

> The best exercises are four that provide the most cardiovascular conditioning: running, swimming, bicycling, and crosscountry skiing. I consider the last the best overall exercise because it can be a total body workout—but you

need snow. Similarly, swimmers need water and bicylists need clear roads. Runners can run almost anywhere, any time, and at a relatively low cost. You can get as many fitness benefits from walking; it just takes a little longer. The best approach may be to combine a number of physical disciplines in an active lifestyle. The triathlon, running, swimming and cycling, is popular. People have discovered that they can do more than one sport.

Comparing Exercises

You can derive different benefits from various forms of exercise. You might like some exercises better than others.

Learn to Walk Again

Although walking is the most natural exercise, many midlife women don't walk enough. Walking may not seem like exercise, but if you walk briskly and often, it is an easy way to gain more vitality and even lose a little weight.
Some other benefits you can derive from walking are:

- Rapid walks for at least 20 minutes five times a week can increase your level of endurance.
- Walking will burn up calories that could otherwise turn to fat.
- Walking will improve the shape of your body by building muscle.
- Building muscle means that you will increase your basal metabolism rate and will burn more calories, even at rest.
- You'll get out of the house and away from food.
- You can have a relaxed time by yourself while out walking.
- Walking is a good time to talk with another person.

According to the Fund for Podiatry Education and Research, there are several basic walking styles, each with different characteristics and benefits.

Strolling

At one or two miles per hour, this is enjoyable but too slow for aerobic or cardiovascular conditioning for the heart and lungs. However, it is a good warmup activity to limber up your body to get ready for more vigorous walking.

Brisk walking

This is aerobic walking, at 3.5 to 5.5 miles per hour. Your pulse stays fairly high for 50 to 60 minutes, and the body burns up 120 to 160 calories per mile.

Long-distance walking

At two to four miles per hour, you'll burn about 100 to 140 calories per mile. Here's how:

- Stride with the longest step comfortable. A long stride stretches and loosens tight muscles. Keep your pace brisk but not hurried. This type of walk increases the amount of oxygen reaching your muscles and brain and leaves you feeling refreshed and exhilarated.
- Walk with your head held high and your back straight; this produces a higher center of gravity and enables you to obtain a longer, more efficient stride.
- With feet two to four inches apart, reach out with hip, knee, and heel, pointing your toes in the direction you are going. A full stride, with knees straight but not locked, and the body column erect, reduces the strain on your back and shoulder muscles.
- Let your arms swing naturally in an arc from your shoulder. This counterbalances your forward motion and increases speed, maintains rhythm, and exercises your upper body.
- Don't tire yourself. If you can't walk for 20 minutes, start with 10 minutes. Increase your time and pace as your body adapts to the exercise.

For additional information on walking, send for a copy of "Walking for Fun and Fitness," a pamphlet published by:

The American Podiatric Medical Association
20 Chevy Chase Circle, N.W.
Washington, D.C. 20015

Running

One 51-year-old women talked with us about the item on our questionnaire regarding exercise:

> Just saying that I exercise regularly more than three times a week doesn't tell you enough about me and what I'd like to share with your readers. I just completed the Chicago ultramarathon. [That means she ran 50 miles.] I don't suggest that all women become long-distance runners, but what I did to get myself in shape for this event—during the menopausal stage of my life—may interest them.

Some people may say that running an ultramarathon is an excess. For me, it's not. I think I do things in moderation, because I do them in stages. I set goals for myself in fitness, relaxation, and stress management.

Being a runner helps me set goals. I don't know which came first, running or setting personal goals. If you want something, you have to figure out how to get there.

I never considered myself an athlete. I was a married schoolteacher with responsibilities of husband, son, and career. During my thirties I began playing tennis several times a week and doing downhill skiing. At age 42 I quit my 25-year smoking habit. I drank quite a bit, too, but stopped.

I started running when I was 44. I couldn't believe how anyone could run a marathon. I ran one mile, then asked myself, "How can I run two miles?" Then I heard about a 10K race [about 6 miles]. I knew one woman who had run in a 10K race, and I thought, "That's the ultimate!" I anticipated that I could probably run four miles, walk one, and crawl the last. I completed the race—running all the way—with bleeding toes the only problem.

Then I began a natural progression. I heard about a half marathon. I trained by increasing two miles every other week. I marked my progress on a calendar for three months. I completed the half marathon. What's necessary is discipline and determination.

After that, she completed seven marathons (26.2 miles each); she ran her first Chicago marathon at age 47. Three of the seven races were in the seven months preceding the 1985 ultramarathon. She was one of two women over age 50 among the ultramarathon runners of whom 147 completed the course: A 54-year-old woman came in seven minutes before her. Sixteen other women from all over the United States, under age 50, also completed the course.

How did I cope with menopausal symptoms? I had irregular periods from age 46 to 50; I'd skip two or three months and then have light and short periods. I had a period the day before one marathon. I stopped having periods when I was 50.

I had hot flashes around the time when I had irregular periods. I'd be on the bus and would get so hot that I had to get off. I couldn't understand how other people could sit there all bundled up. That winter I couldn't wear sweaters or silk blouses.

The hot flashes weren't all. I couldn't sleep at night because of them, or the anticipation of them. I was extremely sensitive to everything that happened around me. I cried a lot. I knew I had to break the pattern.

I went to a doctor who wanted to give me estrogen replacement therapy. I said I'd think about it. My mother died of cancer of the cervix when she was 58. I went to a health food store and asked about alternative therapies. I was advised to take herbal pills for a few weeks; I took hot baths in the evening and set myself up to relax before going to bed. I drank my herbal tea at bedtime.

Within two weeks the hot flashes stopped but I still had irregular periods. Meanwhile, I had a busy, good life at the time, working, running, and participating in an active social life with my husband.

Having my personally set running goals to meet as well as work and family helped me focus on something other than how my declining estrogen supply was affecting me. My mental attitude also helped me cope with the recent loss of my husband.

What is our respondent doing now for a goal, after completing the ultramarathon? "I learned to swim this year. My goal was to do four laps. Now I'm doing one-half mile."

Walking and Aerobic Dancing: Similar Benefits

Midlife women *can* enjoy significant improvements in cardiovascular fitness as a result of participation in aerobic activities, according to a study reported in volume 24 of the *Journal of Sports Medicine* (1984). The journal cited aerobic dancing and walking as resulting in similar improvements in cardiovascular and muscular systems of women aged 50 to 63 after six months of participation. Consistent effort pays off.

Women who are doing aerobic dancing, or are considering starting, should consider several factors:

- A good floor for aerobic dancing provides cushioning as well as stability. Specially built floors in dancing schools are good, as is carpet over heavy padding. Concrete, linoleum, or carpet on concrete may be hazardous.
- Your aerobic dancing shoes should absorb shock, keep your feet stable, and minimize foot twisting. Don't dance barefoot and don't wear runing shoes for dancing. Wear specially designed aerobic dancing shoes.
- Does the program medically screen participants? Some individuals should not begin a program without medical clearance.
- What type of exercise plan does the program follow? The American College of Sports Medicine (ACSM) guidelines suggest three to five exercise sessions per week for 15 to 60 minutes at an intensity of 50% to 90% of maximum heart rate in order to bring about changes in cardiorespiratory efficiency. Programs meeting once a week aren't enough to improve your fitness; for some women, they may be a greater risk than benefit.

- What is the format of the session? It should include a warmup of 5 to 10 minutes, or 15 to 20 minutes for an underexercised woman. The real workout should be from 15 to 60 minutes long. Cool down is necessary. This may be in the form of walking and should gradually slow in pace and last from 5 to 10 minutes. Stretching after exercise may help reduce possible muscle soreness.
- What type of movement or dancing is used? Jerky movements can cause injury and are particularly bad for underexercised women. Avoid programs of this type.
- Is the program progressive? Does it allow enough time for your body to adapt to the training regimen? It may take up to 12 weeks for a training effect to take place.
- The program should include floor work for improving your flexibility, muscular strength, and endurance. Some choreographed programs rely too heavily on the aerobic component with little floor work.
- Don't do any exercises that cause pain. If a step or movement causes you pain, stop doing it.

(This list is adapted from *The Physician and Sportsmedicine*, September 1982 and February 1985.)

Ballroom Dancing

Enough polkas (or folk dancing or dancing to a soft rock beat) can be the equivalent of running a mile. You can use up nine calories a minute in a polka, which is more than the five calories you use in playing golf.

Calisthenics

Be aware that there are some dangers in following calisthenic routines without supervision. Some exercises can be dangerous for certain individuals, particularly to their lower backs. The best way to get into these routines, especially the ones on tapes and records, is to start in a supervised class.

Swimming

While swimming isn't a weight-bearing exercise (weight-bearing exercises help to prevent osteoporosis; see chapters 4 and 5), it can give your muscles and cardiovascular system a good workout. How many calories you use up depends on the stroke and your speed. For example, using the breast stroke will use about 11 calories per minute; with the Australian crawl, about 14 calories per minute.

Swimming is particularly good for overweight individuals because it doesn't put stress on the leg joints and lower back. It is also good for women who have arthritis; some pools have warmer water than usual, just for therapeutic swimming sessions for arthritic patients.

Rope Jumping

You can cut a length of clothesline for a jumping rope. You'll use about the same number of calories in rope jumping as you do in running. However, you may find it difficult to jump rope for as long as you can run (or walk).

Racket Sports

The stop-and-start action of racket sports may help make your legs stronger, and swinging the racket strengthens your chest and shoulder muscles. You use about 10 to 12 calories per minute playing tennis or racketball. You'll use more calories playing singles than doubles. Racket sports may not be advisable for people with certain types of back problems, so consult your doctor first.

Stationary Cycling

You can adjust most stationary bicycles to make the pedaling harder or easier. You can watch the speedometer to see how fast you are going. You'll use up about 11 calories a minute at a speed of 13 miles per hour. (Depending on the tension setting you could use even more.)

Outdoor Bicycling

You'll use the same number of calories outdoors, but may find it more difficult to maintain a steady speed because of traffic and hills.

Rowing Machines

A typical rowing machine will give you an electronic digital readout of your strokes and calories burned per minute. You use about seven calories per minute at a rapid 87 strokes per minute.

Weight-Lifting Machines

Exercise machines require the same amount of muscular energy from the start to the end of a lift, unlike lifting dumbbells. By adjusting knobs or levers on machines, you can increase the strain on your muscles. You can judge your own progress. However, weight-lifting can cause a sudden stress on your heart, which may be dangerous if you have any type of heart disease. Be careful, however; these machines can be dangerous for people with a tendency to slipped discs.

FASHION, COMFORT, AND SAFETY WHILE EXERCISING

There is specially designed wearing apparel for just about any sport you might want to do, from jogging to wind surfing. While such items may be fashionable, you can do most activities comfortably and safely in shorts and a tee shirt, or sweatshirt and sweatpants. Wait to make heavy investments in wearing apparel until you know that you are going to stick with the sport and that special clothing is essential.

However, for comfort and safety, you may want to add some items to your exercise wardrobe, particularly undergarments, protective eyewear, and shoes.

A Firm Foundation

Some women think that vigorous exercise may lead to sagging breasts. Generally, this is not the case, but women with heavy breasts have reported some breast discomfort after jogging or prolonged vigorous activities that cause repeated bouncing.

You can make your breasts and shoulders more comfortable by wearing a specially designed sports bra that supports your breasts and limits their movement more than a regular bra can. Sports bras are usually made of a nonallergenic, nonabrasive, elastized material, such as a blend of cotton and polyester. Wide shoulder straps across the midback decrease chafing. If you have large breasts, you may want to avoid halter-style bras that compress rather than support the breasts in cups.

Protect Your Eyes

If you play racketball or squash, you risk coming in contact with a ball that travels up to 100 miles per hour. Protect yourself by wearing prescription or nonprescription lenses made of industrial safety glass, or plastic mounted into a specially designed frame. Wraparound style eye guards give you wide-angle peripheral vision, which is important in sports.

If you are a tennis player, you will want a less heavy-duty protective device. There are eye guards for individuals who do and do not wear glasses or contact lenses. You can find selections at large sporting goods stores and some eyewear stores and departments.

If you are a swimmer, protect your eyes against irritation caused by chlorinated water or salt water by wearing goggles. You will see better underwater with protective goggles and can avoid bumping into other swimmers and the side of the pool.

Protect Your Feet

If you are a runner, choose a shoe that has adequate cushioning in the midsole, a stable heel cup support to help limit heel movement, and adequate toe space. If you toe in (pronate) or toe out (suppinate), you may want to consult an orthopedist or podiatrist about an orthotic or shoe modification.

Aerobic dancing shoes combine the desirable features of running and court shoes. Specially designed shoes have good reinforcement, good heel and sole cushioning, and a white sole that doesn't leave a scuff mark on the floor.

Tennis and racketball players wear shoes that help push off for quick starts and stops. They have little cushioning in the heel and sole when compared with shoes designed for aerobic dancing or running.

KEEP MOVING

Exercise alone can't change your size and shape. However, exercise, combined with good nutrition and adequate rest, can help you feel better, maintain your ideal weight, and retain your body's natural flexibility. A flexible body moves with ease and grace. You don't have to be a jogger or an aerobic dancer. Just be active on a regular basis and keep your movable parts moving!

8

ENJOY EATING FOR GOOD HEALTH

"In general, mankind, since the improvement of cookery, eats twice as much as nature requires."

Benjamin Franklin, *Poor Richard's Almanac*

"My only real complaint is the weight gain and more matronly midsection I seem to have acquired. I feel it's due to the estrogen. I would love comments on this in your book."

- Does it seem that everything you eat puts weight around your middle?
- Does the fear of overweight interfere with your enjoyment of eating?
- Have you cut down on the quantity you eat and still gain weight?
- If you cut down on quantity, what foods should you include to maintain the most nutritious and enjoyable diet?

If you wonder what you should eat and think you should weigh less, you're not alone. In the Holt-Kahn survey, 11% of the respondents said they were more than 30 pounds overweight and 46.5% said they considered themselves "mildly" overweight. That's over 57% of the group who think they weigh too much!

In this chapter, you'll read about how to maintain your ideal weight, get the most energy from what you eat, choose appropriate foods, and how to determine if you need vitamin and mineral supplements. You'll also read about how to be a successful vegetarian if you want to be, the importance of fiber and water in your diet, the dangers of sodium and sugar, and some tips

141

on taking the worries out of weight control. And, just to add a little spice to this chapter, you'll gain some new cooking tips, which are sprinkled throughout.

WARNING: GOOD DIET MEANS ENJOYMENT, NOT SUFFERING!

This is a chapter about the enjoyment of eating. The word *diet* probably conjures visions of deprivation and suffering. Many midlife women seem to cause themselves undue stress because of concern about their body shapes.

Eating should be a pleasurable experience, not a worrisome one. Eating is a social activity; it's something to do with family, friends, and guests. It's the focus of a party. Eating involves the fun of experimenting with new recipes and surprising those at the table with new dishes. It's fun to try out new cuisines.

Women who cope best with all the other stresses of midlife accept what nature gave them; however, attention to, but not obsession with, your physical shape, and what you put into your body, can help you feel and look better. Because you've had years of experience in meal preparation, you can now put your background to work in making eating more fun and more healthful for yourself, your family, and your guests.

For many, midlife is a time when alterations in cooking habits must be made because of specialized dietary needs beyond just weight control. If you, your husband, or an aging parent develops any of the midlife conditions that require treatment by careful attention to diet, for example, diabetes, heart diseases, or ulcers, you may have to modify recipes accordingly. However, you can apply the same principles of fun and enjoyment about trying out new recipes and a wider variety of foods, and make mealtime fun.

OUR CALORIE-CONSCIOUS GENERATION

We may be the first midlife generation that is so calorie conscious! Look at your family photo albums. Do most of the great-grandmothers and grandmothers stare out at you with content faces and plump shapes?

We are also the first midlife generation that remembers many changes in American eating habits. Perhaps that's why we are still somewhat confused about what is good for us. For example, when we were little, some of our mothers, believing "richer is better," gave us the cream that rose to the top of the milk bottle. Some of our mothers considered baking cookies for us with anything less than all butter serious cruelty to children!

When we were young, many of us gasped with displeasure when we saw fish on the dinner table. The standard of "good diet" in many middle-class American homes for years was a meat-and-potatoes meal almost every night. The habit became particularly ingrained in many families just after World War II, when rationing of meat was discontinued and supplies became plentiful once again.

Then came the revelations about fats and cholesterol being contributors to heart disease. We've cut down on butter and other fats. We've learned that it may be healthier to eat more fish and less meat. We've learned to cook with less salt, because we've heard that too much salt may be bad for our cardiovascular system, particularly if we have high blood pressure. We've encouraged our children to eat less "junk food."

We've learned to modify our diets in many ways that we think are better for us. We've been deluged with diet books, many of which have been national best sellers. Despite all the information, many of us still carry around too many pounds. If any of these diets really worked for many people, would there be a need for a "new" diet each week?

Midlife women are especially conscious of extra weight (as we perceive it) around the midline. Perhaps that's because our American culture has a standard for beauty that finds a sylphlike shape desirable. Thus you may regard your slightest bulges with disdain. But where to cut the calories? You need your milk for calcium and to ward off osteoporosis. You need enough sustenance to give you energy for exercise programs, and if you're not an exerciser, just for everyday life.

WHAT IDEAL WEIGHT AND CALORIES MEAN FOR YOU

You need fewer calories now than when you were younger. Your basal metabolic rate is probably lower, as well as your total energy expenditure. Your basal metabolic rate is the amount of energy it takes to maintain your body at rest. Basal metabolic rates vary among individuals because of differences in body size and composition, physical activity, and endocrine gland activity.

A rough estimate of basal energy needs is:

Ideal weight x 12 = Number of calories needed to maintain the body's metabolic needs.

Example:

120 pounds x 12 = 1,440

A woman whose ideal weight is 120 pounds would require 1,440 calories to maintain her weight. If she consumes more calories, she will have to use them up in exercise or gain weight.

Exercise helps you to lose weight by burning extra calories. But it's been shown that regular exercise can actually increase your basal metabolic rate. In other words, regular exercise will let your body burn calories faster even when you're not exercising. That's why for most people, the combination of exercise and attention to diet is the best plan for controlling weight.

The amount of energy provided by food is described in terms of calories. Your body converts food into energy. The number of calories provided by foods varies based on their protein, carbohydrate, and fat content. You get more calories from fats than from protein and carbohydrates:

1 gram protein	=	4 calories
1 gram carbohydrate	=	4 calories
1 gram fat	=	9 calories

How many calories you need depends on how much energy you burn up. Generally, women need fewer calories than men; women who play a lot of bridge need fewer calories than women who do a lot of jogging. When your body gets extra calories that it doesn't use for energy, it stores them as fat.

You can equate about 1 pound of body fat with about 3,500 calories. Thus, if you eat 500 calories less every day, you will lose one pound in seven days. Or, if you eat 500 extra calories every day, you'll gain a pound in a week.

Some women find it is easier to lose weight by eating larger portions of low-calorie foods and fewer portions of high-calorie foods. If you want to lose weight, consider modifying your diet to include more low-calorie foods.

If you like your present weight, your diet, in terms of calories, is probably appropriate. However, if you want to reduce your weight, there are at least three ways to consider (after an okay from your doctor, of course):

- Eat exactly half of what you eat now (but be sure your nutrient needs are met; i.e., cut out empty calories and seconds).
- Plan your diet according to a calculated daily calorie plan limiting high-calorie foods and including more low-calorie foods.
- Plan your diet according to a daily calorie plan along with a fitness plan.

The third way seems best. Some authorities say weight can be lost by diet alone, or exercise alone, but we believe that the best advice for controlling weight is to consume fewer calories *and* maintain good physical fitness by regular exercise.

GET THE MOST ENERGY FROM WHAT YOU EAT

When you were young, you were told that you had to eat more of certain foods because you were "a growing girl." (Not any more, we hope!) Eating for growth isn't an issue anymore. At midlife, good nutrition must provide necessary elements for your body to function efficiently, repair tissues, and fight off infection.

More importantly, at midlife, your focus should be on nutrient density, or getting as many nutrients as possible for the calories taken in and avoiding "empty calories." By maximizing the opportunities, you can get three or four nutrients from the same food.

Your energy to function efficiently comes from three major sources. You get different benefits from each of these sources:

- Protein
- Carbohydrates
- Fats

Protein

Your body needs protein to maintain your good health. Protein helps build and repair all tissues and your blood. More specifically, protein helps maintain body structure, produce essential compounds, regulate water balance, and provide energy. The best sources of protein are meat, poultry, fish, eggs, milk, and cheese. Other good sources are dried peas and beans, peanut butter, nuts, breads, and cereals.

Since the 1977 Senate Select Committee Report on Nutrition, there has been a popular shift to obtaining protein from poultry and fish instead of red meat. Poultry and fish provide the same essential amino acids as meat but less saturated fat. (See section on fats later in this chapter.)

Carbohydrates

Carbohydrates keep you going. They provide energy and fuel your brain and nervous system. There are two types of carbohydrates: simple and complex.

Simple carbohydrates

Your intestinal tract breaks down simple carbohydrates quickly and easily. Examples of simple carbohydrates are sugar and honey found in such foods as sweet desserts. While you may feel a quick energy lift (or a psychological lift) this type of energy does not stay with you and may leave you feeling even more tired later on. These types of foods provide calories but few if any nutrients.

Complex carbohydrates

These break down more slowly. Examples of foods containing complex carbohydrates are potatoes, pasta, bread, vegetables, and fruits.

A sweet roll contains simple carbohydrates and fat with many calories but few nutrients. When that's all you have for breakfast you get hungry in mid-morning, but if you have a breakfast consisting of an egg, fruit, or whole grain bread, you feel full longer as well as get needed vitamins and minerals.

Nutritionists say you should get 55% of your total calories from complex carbohydrates, no more than 30% from fats, and the remainder from protein. Recently, there have been studies to see whether a very low-fat diet (10%) can prevent cancer and heart disease. The results are not in yet.

Fats

Before menopause, your hormones helped to keep your serum cholesterol low. After menopause, you will lose that protection from estrogen. Now, you can help yourself by reducing the amount of saturated fats you eat before your serum cholesterol rises. Cut down on meat, rich dairy products, and egg yolks. The American Heart Association advises limiting egg yolks to two or three per week.

According to the National Dairy Council, the body needs some fat; all fat is not bad for you. Fat provides some essential nutrients as well as energy, but because of the calories, the fats group is the best place to cut back if you want to lose weight. Also, some fats, primarily the saturated or animal fats, can cause your serum cholesterol to rise, and high cholesterol has been implicated as a risk factor in cardiovascular disease.

Fats are a concentrated source of calories. You get nine calories from each gram of fat, compared with only four calories from a gram of carbohydrate or protein. Many of the foods you eat have hidden fat, such as cottage cheese to which cream has been added. Low-fat milk cottage cheese is available, and has less fat than creamed cottage cheese.

You've heard about three kinds of fat: saturated, polyunsaturated, and monounsaturated. All foods contain carbon, hydrogen, and oxygen in varying amounts. The more carbon, the higher the saturation. Unsaturated fats contain more hydrogen and oxygen. Emphasis should be on unsaturated fats, vegetable oils. Certain fats, such as fish oil and olive oil, may be particularly beneficial.

The United States (along with Finland) has higher death rates from coronary disease than other countries. This has been correlated with a high intake of total fats, cholesterol, and saturated fat. In the mid-1980s, the National Heart, Lung, and Blood Institute convened a cholesterol consensus panel and advocated that dietary recommendations require changing eating habits for all people in the United States over age two! (Start now with your grandchildren!)

The following chart will help you understand the differences between the fats.

Identifying the Fats

Fats	Examples	Characteristics
Saturated	Red meats (beef, pork, lamb, veal) Lard Butter *Palm oil *Coconut oil	Remains solid at room temperature Raises serum cholesterol
Polyunsaturated	Corn oil Safflower oil Vegetable oils (peanut, soybean, cottonseed)	Liquid at cool temperature Helps to lower serum cholesterol
Monounsaturated	**Olive oil Peanut oil	Clouds and thickens slightly when refrigerated Neutral effect on serum cholesterol

*While palm and coconut oil are plant oils, they are saturated fat because of their chemical composition.

**Olive oil is another exception. It has a different chemical composition than other plant oils.

CHOOSE APPROPRIATE FOODS

The "basic four" food groups you learned about in school haven't changed. What has changed is our understanding of how to use the food groups for the best possible health benefits.

The "basic four" are:

- Fruits and vegetables.
- Breads and cereals.
- Milk, cheese, and dairy products.
- Meat, poultry, fish, and beans.

Fruits and Vegetables

Almost all fruits and vegetables are low in fat and contain no cholesterol. They are "nutrient dense" and contain few calories. You can enjoy fruits and vegetables as snacks throughout the day.

Consider a typical portion as one piece or one-half cup. For example, one orange, the juice of one lemon, one medium potato, or one-half cup of cooked vegetable. You should include one good source of Vitamin C, such as a citrus fruit or juice every day. Other good sources are also deep yellow or dark green vegetables, and unpeeled fruits and vegetables, and those with edible seeds, such as berries.

Fruits and vegetables are important sources of various vitamins, minerals, and fiber. Different foods in this group vary by fiber and nutrient content. Choose a variety of foods to provide the total of vitamins and minerals required for good health.

Dark green and deep yellow vegetables are good sources of Vitamin A. Most dark green vegetables, when not overcooked, and citrus fruits (oranges, grapefruit, tangerines, lemons), melons, berries, and tomatoes are also good sources of Vitamin C and folic acid (folacin). Dark green vegetables are good sources of riboflavin (Vitamin B$_2$), folacin, iron, and magnesium. Some greens, most notably collards, kale, mustard, turnips, and dandelion, and broccoli, contain calcium.

Fruits, particularly oranges and bananas, are important sources of potassium. Women taking some medications—for example, thiazide diuretics—need extra potassium.

To preserve the color and texture of vegetables, steam them in a basket-type steamer. When they are just barely done, run cold water over them to stop the cooking.

Breads and Cereals

There's been a change in attitude about bread in past 10 years. Years back, we thought carbohydrates, such as bread, potatoes, and noodles, were fattening, and we considered these foods "no-no's" if we hoped to control our weight. Now nutritionists recommend that 55% of our total caloric intake should come from complex carbohydrates (bread, potatoes, pasta, vegetables, and fruits).

Pasta, potatoes, bread, and rice provide good sources of B Vitamins, which midlife women need, and fiber. These foods also help us to feel satisfied after a meal and to stay regular.

For breads and cereals, consider a typical portion as one slice of bread, one-half to two-thirds cup of cooked cereal, noodles, or rice. You should include four servings of these foods each day. This group includes products made with whole grains or enriched flour or meal, such as bread, muffins, cooked or ready-to-eat cereals, cornmeal products, noodles, rice, oats, barley, and bulgur.

Whole grain and enriched foods are important sources of the B Vitamins, provide some protein, and contain more fiber than most processed grain products.

Commercially prepared breakfast cereals come "fortified" with nutrients. Natural whole grain cereals are preferable to sugarcoated, fortified cereals. Some fortified cereals contain vitamins not usually found in cereals, such as Vitamins A, B_{12}, C, and D. If you have a balanced diet, you don't need to obtain these vitamins from "enriched" cereals; you will get them from other foods in your diet.

Good cereals are cooked oatmeal and farina made with the whole grain. Avoid instant hot cereals that are loaded with sugar.

Milk and Cheese

Midlife is not the time to skimp on dairy products to save calories. Cut down on your consumption of soft drinks and drink more milk (if you can) to increase your calcium intake. Soft drinks contain phosphates that may actually inhibit the absorption of the calcium from the milk you do consume.

Select low-fat, low-salt milk-group foods so that you get the most nutrients without the calories. You have a choice of whole, skim, low-fat, buttermilk, evaporated, and nonfat dry milk; also yogurt, ice milk, ice cream, cheese, and cottage cheese. An eight-ounce cup of milk is one serving. Usual portions of commonly used dairy products and their milk equivalents in calcium are:

1 cup plain yogurt	=	1 cup milk
1/2 cup ice cream or ice milk	=	1/3 cup milk
1/2 cup cottage cheese	=	1/4 cup milk
1 inch cube Cheddar or Swiss cheese	=	1/2 cup milk

After reading the chapters on osteoporosis, you understand why your needs for foods from the milk and cheese group are higher now than when you were younger. Young adults need two servings each day, and menopausal and postmenopausal women should have four servings. Consume foods from the milk and cheese group with high calcium but lower caloric values, such as yogurt instead of cottage cheese, or frozen yogurt instead of ice cream.

Remember that you can count the milk you use in cooked foods, such as creamed soups and puddings, toward your daily quota.

Milk and most milk products are the major source of calcium in the American diet. Also, you get riboflavin, Vitamins A, B_6 and B_{12}, and Vitamin D from your fortified milk products. Examples of such fortified products are low-fat or skim milk products that have the nutrients of whole milk products but fewer calories. Don't overlook other low-fat, high-protein foods, such as tofu.

Meat, Poultry, Fish, and Beans

Meat is an important source of heme iron (a form of iron that has the hemoglobin that enables your blood cells to carry oxygen) that helps keep your blood rich. Meat, poultry, and fish are all good sources of protein. Select lean cuts of beef, pork, and lamb. Bake, broil, or poach instead of frying.

Consider 2 to 3 ounces (without bone) of lean, cooked meat, poultry, or fish a serving. One egg, 1/2 to 3/4 cup of cooked dry beans, dry peas, or lentils; 2 tablespoons of peanut butter, and 1/4 to 1/2 cup of nuts, sesame seeds, or sunflower seeds count as one ounce of meat, poultry, or fish. You should have two servings each day from this basic group.

Foods in this group are high in protein, phosphorus, and Vitamins B_6, B_{12}, and others. Vary your choices among these foods because different foods contain different nutritional benefits. For example, only foods of animal origin contain B_{12} naturally. Red meats and oysters contain zinc. Liver and egg yolks contain Vitamin A, but are also high in dietary cholesterol. Dry peas, soybeans, and nuts contain magnesium.

Most fish and poultry are relatively low in calories and saturated fat, compared to prime cuts of beef, pork, or lamb. Seeds, such as sunflower or sesame, and walnuts and legumes contain polyunsaturated fatty acids. Avoid bacon, sausages, luncheon meats, and hot dogs. Fat often makes up 80% of the calories in processed meats.

You can make the dishes you prepare lower in fat, too. For example, when you make soups, a meat stew with vegetables, or chili, let the dish chill overnight (or all day long) in the refrigerator. Remove the fat that solidifies at the top.

Fats, Sweets, and Alcohol

After the basic four food groups, there's another group that includes foods such as butter, margarine, mayonnaise, candy, jams, jellies, soft drinks, wine, beer, and liquor. Some of these foods appear as ingredients in prepared foods or are added to other foods at the table. Most bakery products are also in this group because they contain relatively low levels of vitamins, minerals, and protein compared with calories.

There is no recommended number of daily servings suggested from this group; none are nutritionally necessary. How many servings you eat with a clear conscience depends on the number of calories you require to maintain your ideal weight. You get calories from these items, and little else. Vegetable oil, however, does provide Vitamin E and essential fatty acids. A small amount of fat is needed in your diet; however, most Americans eat more dietary fat than necessary. Unsaturated fats such as corn and olive oil are in general less damaging to the cardiovascular system.

Alcohol has 7 calories per gram, and the higher a beverage's alcoholic content, the more calories it has. Alcohol has no known nutritional value and is considered an "empty calorie" beverage. However, one or two ounces of alcohol per day may help protect against cardiovascular disease.

In the Holt-Kahn survey, in response to the question "Do you drink alcohol?" 13% said none, 58.8% said "occasional drink," 21.7% said one or two drinks per day, and 5.1% said more than two drinks per day.

VITAMINS AND MINERALS

In the survey, 60.6% of all respondents said they take vitamins; 36.3% said they do not (the rest didn't answer this question).

Should you take vitamin supplements? "Not if you have a well-balanced diet," says Linda V. Van Horn, Ph.D., R.D., spokesperson for the American Dietetic Association and Associate Professor, Department of Community Health and Preventive Medicine, Northwestern University School of Medicine, Northwestern University, Chicago. "However, if your lifestyle doesn't allow you to shop, prepare food, and eat regular servings of many appropriate foods, you may want to take a simple, multiple vitamin with iron. But don't take megadoses of a single vitamin or mineral," she cautions. "Foods are the best source of vitamins because they are more likely to be bioavailable or absorbed more effectively. Vitamins work synergistically. For example, Vitamin D, calcium, and phosphorus are absorbed best when they are consumed in the proper balance, as found in milk. If you think you need calcium supplements, your best chance of absorption occurs if they are taken with milk. Milk offers the best opportunity for calcium and other nutrients to work together."

The following section will give you a review of what vitamins do for you, some guidelines to help you know if you are getting enough, and some tips on how to prepare your foods to conserve the most vitamin content.

What are vitamins? They aren't just alphabet soup! They are a mixture of chemicals necessary to regulate various body processes, to aid the metabolism of protein and carbohydrates, and to give you energy.

Some vitamins are water soluble; others are fat soluble.

Water-Soluble Vitamins

Water-soluble vitamins are not stored in the body. In serving and cooking, they can be destroyed by air or steam. The most helpful water-soluble vitamins are C and the B Vitamins (including niacin).

Vitamin C

Citrus fruits are the best sources of Vitamin C, also known as ascorbic acid. Other good sources are strawberries, cantaloupe, tomatoes, peppers, potatoes, cabbage, broccoli, and greens. To get the maximum Vitamin C content, eat fruits as soon after they are picked as possible. Keep fruit juices in covered containers in your refrigerator.

B vitamins

These include B_1 (thiamine), niacin, B_6 (pyroxidine) and B_{12}. Good sources are eggs, wheat germ, liver, pork, green peas, and beans. You need B_6 for hemoglobin synthesis and B_{12} for red blood cell formation.

You get B_2 (riboflavin) from eggs, pork, beef, spinach, liver, milk, and cheese. Riboflavin deficiency can lead to extreme sensitivity to light, reddened lips, and cracks around the corners of the mouth.

You get B_6 (pyroxidine) from meats, vegetables, and whole grain cereals. Deficiency can lead to anemia, weakness, neuritis, and sores at the corners of the mouth and/or eyes.

You get B_{12} from meats, fruits, vegetables, and dairy products. Deficiency of B_{12} can lead to pernicious anemia; this vitamin is necessary to bring red blood cells to maturity.

You get niacin in red meat, yeast, milk, and fresh vegetables. A deficiency results in pellagra, a disease that was fairly prevalent in the United States in the early 1900s.

Fat-Soluble Vitamins

Fat-soluble vitamins are A, D, E, and K. You store them in your body and absorb them with dietary fats.

You get Vitamin A (retinol) from green leafy vegetables, carrots, dairy products, eggs, some fish, and fish liver oils. A symptom of extreme Vitamin A deficiency is night blindness.

You get Vitamin D from fortified milk, fish oil, eggs, and exposure to sunlight. You need Vitamin D for calcium metabolism. Rickets (a softening of the bones) is a disease that results from a shortage of calcium, phosphorus, or Vitamin D. You can develop a deficiency of Vitamin D from overuse of laxatives because too frequent elimination may deplete these minerals and vitamins.

You get Vitamin E (tocopherol) from green leafy vegetables and seeds. Some health food retailers promote literature that claims that Vitamin E reduces arterial blood clots, relieves sterility, and helps hair grow. These claims are *not* well founded or well accepted by nutritionists.

You get Vitamin K (phylloquinone) from green leafy vegetables and small amounts in cereals, fruits, and meats. Vitamin K is important in forming the substances that enable your blood to clot properly.

What About Minerals?

Minerals are also necessary for your body to function efficiently. Minerals help develop and maintain your teeth, bones, and chemical reactions. With a balanced diet, that is, some foods from each group every day, you will get enough of the essential minerals: calcium, phosphorus, iron, and iodine. You get these from milk products, including cheese; green leafy vegetables; fish; and liver. Iodine is not found in many foods, but is included in many processed and packaged foods in the form of iodized salt. If you do use salt on the table or in cooking, use iodized salt.

You get phosphorus from protein-rich foods; phosphorus is necessary in combination with calcium for strong bones and teeth. About 90% of phosphorus comes in combination with calcium.

Many minerals are essential in minute quantities. An example is copper, which helps the body make iron into hemoglobin for the blood. Another is fluorine, which helps prevent tooth decay. Some drinking water supplies are fortified with fluorine.

ARE YOU A VEGETARIAN?

You *can* be a healthy vegetarian at any age. However, you must remember to combine your incomplete proteins to derive the best nutritional values from the foods you eat.

If you are a lacto-ovo vegetarian (eat milk and eggs plus vegetables, fruits, and grains), you will have less trouble getting enough protein and iron than a strict vegetarian (no animal products, only fruits, vegetables, and grains). Strict vegetarians, however, are usually highly motivated and know enough about nutrition so that they can derive enough nutrients without depleting their reserves. Any person on a vegetarian diet who does not feel well and suspects that a depeletion of minerals, etc., is occurring should see a physician.

An individual with a lactose intolerance can be a successful lacto-vegetarian. Lact-aid added to milk hydrolyzes lactose and prevents the untoward side effects of lactose ingestion. Lactose-free soy milks are available. Most lactose-intolerant persons tolerate cheese well.

FIBER

Fiber is the part of plant food, such as fruits, vegetables, and grains, that does not break down during digestion; thus it is not specifically a nutrient. Dietary fiber, however, aids the efficient functioning of your digestive tract. You can help prevent constipation by having a sufficient amount of fiber in your diet every day. Fiber helps retain water in your intestines, adds bulk to stools and softens them, and regulates the time it takes for food waste to move through your body.

Fiber in your diet is preferable to laxatives. Frequent use of laxatives can reduce your body's ability to function on its own. Some laxatives can lead to loss of fluids and essential minerals.

Add fiber to your diet by eating more whole grain breads and cereals, fresh fruits, raw vegetables, and nuts. The key words to remember are raw and rough. Retain fiber in the foods you cook by steaming, not boiling, them. Fibrous foods are also important to give you a feeling of satiety after a meal.

Nutrition researchers are actively looking at the role of fiber in the American diet. For example, one project underway in the Department of Community Health and Preventive Medicine at Northwestern University's School of Medicine in Chicago involves the role of water-soluble fiber found in oats in reducing serum cholesterol.

Elsewhere, another project involves looking at the possibility of eliminating the need for insulin by some insulin-dependent diabetics by use of a high-fiber diet. Some researchers have found that fiber reduces after-meal blood glucose levels. It is hypothesized that fiber may improve the ability of some cells to receive and use insulin. Several studies have indicated that a high-fiber diet might reduce the risk of colon cancer.

DRINKING WATER FOR BETTER HEALTH

Drinking plenty of fluids is essential for your good health and fitness. Nutrition experts advise drinking six to eight glasses each day. You need more if you exercise heavily, or are in a hot climate and perspire heavily.

Water facilitates all the chemical reactions in your body. It helps carbohydrates, proteins, and fats release energy and expedites movement of nutrients. All the water you consume need not be just from drinking liquids. There is water in many of the foods you eat, especially fruits and vegetables (lettuce is 95% water).

SODIUM

As the generation that grew up and matured along with the convenience food industry, we have become accustomed to eating many foods that have been processed with large quantities of salt. "Since the early 1900s, we're eating as much as 10 times more sodium than we need," says Dr. Van Horn.

Some say salt, some say sodium. The chemical name is sodium chloride. It is about 40% sodium and 60% chloride by weight. Sodium helps regulate your blood pressure and the volume of your blood, controls the amount of fluid around your body's cells, and is necessary for the contraction of your heart and other muscles and for relaying nerve impulses. Chloride controls water flow across cell walls, aids digestion, and helps keep the blood chemically balanced.

You get sodium in your diet from many sources. Some foods have more sodium content than others; examples are milk, fish, and meats. Fresh fruits and most vegetables are relatively low in natural sodium.

According to the National Research Council and the U. S. Dept. of Agriculture, one teaspoon of salt contains about 2,000 milligrams of sodium. A "safe and adequate sodium intake per day is about 1,000 to 3,300 milligrams for an adult." Estimates are that the average American adult consumes between 2,300 and 6,900 milligrams of sodium each day.

During the last decade, the role of salt as a contributor to high blood pressure has been extensively researched. First it was clearly implicated as a culprit, and persons with high blood pressure and other cardiovascular diseases were put on low-salt or salt-restricted diets. Then some researchers suggested that salt may not be a factor for many individuals. The controversy continues, but is heavily weighted in favor of a low-salt diet.

Excess fluid retention is a complaint many women have while menstruating and after menopause. Salt aggravates retention of body fluids. Excess body fluid plays a role in premenstrual syndrome and menstrual discomfort and causes feelings of bloating and other annoyances for many women of all ages.

You can eliminate many minor symptoms by reducing your salt intake. Preference for salty taste is learned, and you can learn to change your behavior. You can't do yourself any harm by reducing your salt intake, and you are likely to do yourself good.

Some helpful hints:

- Take your salt shaker off the table.
- Avoid foods naturally high in sodium (olives, pickles, condiments).
- Avoid foods with "visible" salt, such as potato chips and pretzels.
- Limit your intake of some canned and frozen products that have high salt content, such as tomato juice, tomato paste, canned vegetables, and some frozen dinners.
- Check the labels of all processed, canned, or boxed foods for sodium content. Choose those that indicate a low- or no-salt or sodium content.

- Cut down on canned soups and sauces. Instead, for example, make your own basic soup stock. You'll cut down on the fat as well as the sodium content.

SUGAR AND ARTIFICIAL SWEETENERS

Sugar, like alcohol, is an empty-calorie food. You get sugar in many foods, including baked goods, which may also be high in fat content. Craving sweets, like craving salty foods, is a learned behavior. If you are a sweet-craver, try retraining yourself to enjoy dried or fresh fruit in place of cookies, pies, or cakes for dessert. You can get the satisfaction of having a sweet, as well as some minerals, from changing your habit.

Although artificial sweeteners cut down on calories when used instead of sugar, they provide the sweetness to which you may have become accustomed. While you are changing your eating behavior, you can also retrain your palate and cut down on use of artificial sweeteners. "The jury is still out on the long range effects of artificial sweeteners, especially on the quantity issue," says Dr. Van Horn. "A little bit won't hurt most people. However, the combined effect of artificial sweeteners in soft drinks, jelly, and other foods, could be harmful to some individuals, so it's best to just restrict your total amount to be safe," she advises.

THE SHAPE IN WHICH YOU LIVE

You need a commitment to consistency to keep your body in the shape in which you like to live. Nutritionists advise that maintaining ideal weight is the healthiest situation for most midlife women. Eating patterns are part of your lifestyle. You don't start on day 1 and stop on day 30, even though your currently popular diet may say so. Your eating habits should be lifelong.

If you have been on weight loss diets at various times and are still more than 10 pounds overweight, you probably haven't learned very much from those diets. If your weight fluctuates up and down, the "Yo-Yo" effect may represent an eating problem.

If you want to control your weight:

- Don't shop on an empty stomach. If you go to the grocery store hungry, you may make unnecessary purchases.
- Eat more slowly.
- Prepare smaller portions.
- Avoid "seconds."

- Change your eating habits by becoming aware of your own eating problems.
- Keep a "food diary." Write down:
  - What you ate
  - Time of day (e.g., lunch, mid-afternoon, late evening, etc.)
  - Reason for eating at that time (e.g., dinner, lonesome, tired, angry, etc.)

After keeping your diary for a few days, you may begin to see a pattern. For example, you may find that on days when you skip breakfast, you eat a sweet roll in mid-morning; and on days when you eat breakfast, you are satisfied with no mid-morning snack and only a salad for lunch. You may find that controlling your appetite is easier all day long if you start the day with breakfast.

However, if you are an individual who isn't hungry at breakfast time, eat your early meal later. Call it brunch, but don't overeat and then go the rest of day without eating anything else. The important new pattern to establish is eating several small meals each day on a regular basis.

Eating because of loneliness may be a more difficult situation to alter. However, being aware of using eating as a coping mechanism is a start. Call a friend. Join a new community group. If you are active, you'll be less likely to reach for food between meals. Join a support group and learn how other people cope. Your food diary will help keep you aware of why you eat too much.

If you eat compulsively because of anger toward yourself or others, family tensions, marital or sexual problems, lack of a partner, boredom, or loneliness, read Geneen Roth's book, *Feeding the Hungry Heart*. You'll learn how others recognize, deal with, and resolve the compulsion to eat.

Can you be too thin? Not according to the pictures in the fashion magazines! However, being too thin can cause a lack of energy. Individuals who are excessively thin may not be meeting their nutritional needs. They may have a depressed immune response, and won't have the reserves of energy needed to fight off infection.

It may reassure you, and the 56% of the respondents in our survey who consider themselves overweight, that long-term studies show that it is healthier to be slightly (not more than 5 pounds) overweight than underweight.

Some psychiatrists say that eating disorders, such as bulimia and anorexia, are on the increase among midlife women. Bulimia is the "binge and purge" pattern. Anorexia is self-imposed starvation to achieve thinness. Both patterns are unhealthy and should be treated by a physician.

Some people experience a natural loss of appetite as they age. However, with a little extra exercise, their basal metabolic rate will increase, appetite may increase, and, consequently, their energy level will increase, and they will feel better.

Eating is one of the joys of life. It's one way of sharing with others. It's the focus of many holidays and parties. And it's fun to experiment with new foods. Become more flexible in your attempts to control your weight, and have some fun! Enjoy eating for good health!

9

WHAT'S "ALL IN YOUR HEAD"?

"The pictures are all hung, the children gone. It's time to think not of what might be, but what is. You look not at what might be about your spouse, your job, yourself, but at what you have. If you can live with it, fine. If you can't, it's your last chance to change and build a new life."

"I'd like to see some discussion of mental attitudes toward menopause. A lot of women talk themselves into depression. Active and busy women—mentally and physically—are not downed by this change in their bodies."

"How much is in my head, and how much is menopause?"

There has always been confusion about which changes of midlife for women are physical and which are due to external social changes. Physical changes include:

- Gradual or rapid fluctuation of estrogen and progesterone with eventual fall in levels
- Increases in pituitary hormones LH and FSH
- Increasing proportion of adrenal hormones, which can have male hormone-type side effects
- Gradual decrease in metabolic rate
- Loss of skin and muscle tone

Social changes that may occur at this time include:

- Loss of youthful image in a youth-oriented culture.
- Loss of maternal role.

- For some, loss of spouse or other partner due to widowhood or divorce; lack of new partner.
- Plateauing in career track or having to start fresh after years out of the job market.
- Physical ailments start to replace the health and energy taken for granted by the young.

Which changes are physical? Which changes are emotional? Can you separate the two? Several hints stand out from the responses to the Holt-Kahn survey:

- Women who have a good self-concept and rewarding roles in life suffer fewer physical symptoms of menopause.
- Women whose self-esteem is based on things that are changing in negative ways are likelier to suffer severe symptoms.
- Many women who find themselves depressed, irritable, and "out of control" feel much better on hormone therapy. At times, women whose physical problems are improved by estrogen replacement therapy feel better about themselves.

What these factors point to is a complicated interaction between physical, mental, and social changes. Like puberty, menopause occurs at a time when our social roles and position in society may be changing at the same time our bodies are in a state of flux. Such rapid changes can be unsettling and confusing.

Here are some examples of how women have felt, based on true stories.

JOAN

Joan W. is a 51-year-old mother of three who has been actively involved in volunteer work and entertaining for her husband, who is a successful attorney. After their youngest child left for college, Joan's husband announced that he wanted a divorce. Joan retained the house, but found she could not afford to keep it up or heat it. Gradually, the house sank into disarray. Joan's friends drifted away from her because their activities were mainly couple-oriented. When Joan found herself fearful of leaving the house, her daughter insisted that she enter the hospital psychiatric unit.

Gradually, Joan came to realize that she had depended on outer role definitions to feel good about herself. Deprived of her wife/mother role, she had little to fall back on.

Today, Joan lives in a modest apartment and works as a sales clerk, a role for which she feels overeducated, but she realizes her college English major won't get her much of a job. She is taking word-processing courses and hopes to get an administrative assistant job soon. She feels very bitter about the breakup of her marriage and her husband's new life with a young, now-pregnant wife. She is even more bitter because she feels she wasted the years she devoted to him when she could have been developing her own skills and interests.

MARY

Mary M. is also 51. She also raised three children. While her children were small, she did home sewing and tailoring for friends. Ten years ago, she opened her own tailoring shop, despite gentle kidding from her husband about her "Ladies' Sewing Circle." Today her store has four full-time employees and sells fabrics, runs sewing classes, and has an interior design consulting business. Her husband, pleasantly surprised at the store's financial success, made a midlife change from selling insurance to personal financial consulting, which pays less but in which he is far happier. In the midst of this success, one of their sons died of a drug overdose. She and her husband drew closer together and resolved their grief through church activities and volunteering with local parents' groups.

Does this seem like the stuff of soap operas? These are both real-life dramas and illustrate two major points about midlife. One is that women who have several roles based on their own talents will fare better against the setbacks life deals us all. You will have fewer setbacks if your roles are multiple and if you feel good about yourself. If you don't, it's time to start changing!

> "I'd like to see a detailed explanation of mood swings, how to control them, how to prepare for aging and acceptance of aging. I'd like to see healthy attitudes rather than bitterness at aging."

> "Do something to dispel the myth that women after menopause are worthless."

Midlife has its share of stresses. Women who experience natural menopauses usually are at an age of significant and sometimes critical psychological and social changes. These key life issues are unrelated to the women's physiological or endocrine status. Sometimes it is hard to sort out feelings caused by typical midlife issues and those caused by a failing estrogen supply.

MIDLIFE STRESSES ARE REAL

Certain scenarios disturb many women:

- Facing an empty nest
- Realizing that you won't have any more children to mother
- Knowing that your body has changed and that you may not be as "attractive" as you once were in a culture that has for women equated youth with beauty
- Moving from a larger home to a smaller one, possibly in another area
- Helping your husband or another loved one deal with a major illness
- Helping your husband or another loved one cope with *his* midlife development
- Coping with sexual problems because of vaginal dryness and/or changes in male physiology
- Facing social and economic consequences of divorce or widowhood
- Missing a sex life because of the lack of a partner
- Seeking a new partner and adjusting to a second marriage and a set of second-hand problems with another's children or parents
- Dealing with aging parents
- Contemplating your own old age
- Reentering the career world
- Seeking out meaningful volunteer activities

At midlife, women ask themselves: What have I done with my life? Where am I going from here? How they feel about themselves depends on their responses.

THE "EMPTY NEST"

"It was not an empty nest. I was tickled that the children could be on their own. That was my job, to train them to be self-sufficient, to work myself out of the mothering job. I've found that once a mother, always a mother. It's just a more mature relationship. Their problems are their problems. And they've solved some real tough ones on their own."

"I'm furious at psychologists who talk about the empty nest syndrome. Most of us would love to be living our own lives without still worrying about the hang-on adult latchkey kids and their problems."

Happy midlife women assess what they've done and look at their grown children with pride and a sense of accomplishment. Many women begin to plan their lives around new options now open to them. They now make more decisions themselves and learn to do more things for themselves. They become more autonomous, particularly if they are widowed or divorced.

The "empty nest" syndrome, as a stressful factor during midlife, seems to affect women less during the late 1980s than ever before. Some women find it a tremendous relief to have their children grown up and away from home. Many women who have matured during the women's movement look at release from children positively. They don't approach the change in status with a feeling of worthlessness.

Women who continue a good relationship with their children, in-laws, and grandchildren, and those whose identity is less child-centered, are less stressed when their children enter the adult world. Many find more satisfaction from their marriage—or a sense of freedom if they are now single—when grown children leave home.

However, among women for whom the empty nest is accompanied by dissolution of a marriage or poor health (either her own or her spouse's), or other problems, the situation becomes more difficult to sort out.

MOOD SWINGS AND HORMONES

"Face lifts may make some women feel better. Physical changes are natural, in her and him. Accept yourself. That's part of self-esteem."

"I had a hysterectomy and my ovaries removed at age 48. I was instantly menopausal. I am an even-tempered person. I'm a mental health professional and recognized that I was going through a manic-depressive cycle ten times a day. After two weeks, the gynecologist said that I shouldn't have waited that long and should have called. He prescribed Premarin tablets. I take it 21 days a month. I feel normal. I can't bleed because I have no uterus. I have the best of all possible worlds."

Some women who feel unable to cope with daily stresses associated with midlife and hormonal changes go to their physicians with complaints of mood swings, irritability, and fatigue. Some women ask for estrogen because they believe it will help them feel better. Many physicians reinforce this notion and prescribe estrogen replacement therapy without investigating the coincidental issues women face.

Are mood swings related to hormonal levels, or do they result from changing attitudes of self-image? There is controversy over the effects of estrogen on psychological well-being.

"I believe mood swings, including depression and manic feelings, are about half-hormonal and half-psychological," says Phyllis Perlman, R.N., nurse-psychotherapist, Bayshore, New York: "When estrogen levels decrease, there are definite mood changes. I don't know where one begins and one ends. However, if women had a poor self-image before, they are likely to have a harder time during menopause. Around menopause, many focus on their no-longer youthful bodies. After menopause, I've noticed that many of my patients achieve a more peaceful state of mind. They find their niche in the world and their hormonal changes have calmed down."

Before taking estrogen replacement therapy for anything less than debilitating physical symptoms, consider your state of mind. How are you dealing with the stresses and options you face? How can you know if your responses are appropriate and healthy? If you don't like the way you feel, what can you do to feel better?

SELF-EXAM FOR YOUR OWN HEAD

We've been taught about self-examinations. We do breast self-exams routinely. Some feminist women's health centers teach women to do their own vaginal and pelvic exams. Now it's time to do a self-examination of your midlife head. This is something all women can and should do!

For the following questions, rate yourself on a scale of 1 though 10. A 10 is tops; 1 is the pits. See the interpretation of your score at the end of the following list of questions.

	No	Sometimes	Yes
	1	5	10

Do I feel good about myself?
Do I like the way I look?
Am I pleased with my weight?
Do I compliment myself often?
Is my appetite good?
Do I sleep all right most of the time?
Do I handle anger appropriately when
   things bother me?
Am I with other people as much as I
   like to be?
Do I think other people are as good as I
   am?
Do I think other people are supportive of
   me and my efforts?

	No	Sometimes	Yes
	1	5	10

Married women: Is my marital relationship good?

Are my social relationships good?

Is my sex life satisfying?

Is my relationship with my children good?

If parents are alive, is my relationship with them good?

If they are deceased, I have no regrets about unresolved conflicts with them.

Do I enjoy my favorite activities as much as I did a few years ago?

Do I derive pleasure from a variety of activities?

Am I free from addiction to alcohol and drugs?

Scoring Yourself

If your answers average 5 or above, you're probably feeling okay. If your answers hover much under 5, and you say to yourself that you don't like being this way, you may want to look carefully at factors that you can change for the better. You can change many of your attitudes yourself. Or you may want to seek the help of a special-interest support group or a trained therapist.

STOP DEPRESSING YOURSELF

> "Depression is insidious. I regret not recognizing it sooner as possibly menopausal. The last five-year-period has been the pits emotionally. I'm 55 now."

> "I'd like to see ideas on how to manage fluctuating emotions. I'm often angry about something, which is not my usual self."

We all feel blue or down once in a while. It's perfectly normal to feel that way at times. We live in an imperfect world and things don't always go right.

Feeling up or down is closely connected to self-esteem, or how you feel about yourself. "Depression is related to anger turned against yourself in terms of disappointment and resentment about events that have happened," explains Gabrielle Woloshin, M.D., a Highland Park, Illinois, psychiatrist in midlife herself. "Anger toward oneself takes many forms. For example, some women think that they didn't do what they were supposed to do with their lives, or that their children didn't turn out as well as they might have. Recognizing and acknowledging these kinds of regrets makes them less stressful."

If you have ongoing or frequent periods of feeling down, think about what you do to depress yourself. Ask yourself what you can do about it. Here are some ideas:

- Get more support from friends
- Take a course, take up an activity, just to please yourself
- Develop new goals for yourself, in work, exercise, sports, education, or hobbies
- Find additional avenues for gratification
- Do something to get what you want rather than complain about an existing situation

If you've tried these ideas and they haven't worked for you, or you still don't feel better, if every day is a gray one and you feel as though you're in a black hole, you may benefit from professional help.

How Mental Health Professionals Diagnose and Treat Depression

Typical ongoing symptoms of depression are:

- Profound sadness
- Loss of appetite or overeating
- Sleep disturbances such as trouble falling asleep, trouble waking up, or waking up too early
- No enjoyment or pleasure from previously pleasurable activities
- Lethargy and chronic forgetfulness
- A feeling of "being stuck" and "not being able to get going"
- Being stalled in a phase of mourning
- Constant self-criticism

There is a group of disorders, referred to by mental health workers as "affective disorders" or "mood disorders."

According to the American Psychiatric Association's *Diagnostic and Statistical Manual*, "The essential feature of this group of disorders is a disturbance of mood, accompanied by a full or partial manic or depressive syndrome, that is not due to any other physical or mental disorder. Mood refers to a prolonged emotion that colors the whole psychic life; it generally involves either depression or elation."

These problems are treated with psychotherapy, and, in some cases, medication. Appropriate cases respond dramatically to specific medications. Medications that affect moods are known as psychotropic medications, and their use must be carefully monitored and controlled by a physician.

Many mood disorders respond best to a relationship with an interested and impartial professional.

GETTING PROFESSIONAL HELP

> *"A positive attitude and relaxation and easement of stress are helpful. I forced myself to do many things when staying at home would have been easier. Now I am happy I did. Menopause comes when we have other problems, too. Professional help can be wonderful. For example, I worried so about my father until a psychiatrist helped me realize that there was little I could do."*

Where to Go for Help

If you think that you can't cope with your emotional swings and feelings of low self-esteem and want to get help, you need to share these feelings either with an understanding friend or with a professional counselor. There are many types of therapists in the helping professions.

You might want to choose a therapist who is personally recommended by a friend. Or you may not want to talk with your friends about your need for emotional therapy. In that case, consider asking your family physician, internist, or gynecologist for a recommendation.

If the first therapist you see does not seem a good "fit" with your personality and needs, find another one. When choosing any kind of therapist, check out credentials. Know whether your therapist is a psychiatrist, psychologist, or psychiatric social worker. Find out where the therapist received his or her training, and check with that institution. Also, there are professional societies for many specialties. Check with an appropriate organization to see that your therapist has the accreditation to counsel in your community.

When to seek an M.D. therapist for an emotional problem

If you've tried going to a non-M.D. regarding some of your symptoms and haven't found relief, maybe you should consult an M.D. Also, you'll want an M.D. if:

- You need medication. M.D.s are the only mental health therapists who can prescribe medications. For certain emotional illnesses, medications are helpful.

- You have incapacitating or debilitating symptoms.
- You have other medical problems for which you are receiving care and medication.
- There is a history of mental illness in your family, other family members have ever been hospitalized for mental illness, or you require hospitalization for a mental problem.

When to seek a non-M.D. therapist for an emotional problem

Good mental health is a continuum. If you recognize what your problems are and just have occasional periods of feeling sorry for yourself, you probably don't need therapy by a psychiatrist. You also probably don't need a psychiatrist if:

- The end of your problem is in sight, but you just can't seem to get there by yourself.
- You realize your symptoms are of short duration and you can identify the stress that brought them on.

Clinics often have all the above and a sliding scale for payment, and may be helpful in assisting you in your decision about which kind of professional will best meet your needs. Support groups may be helpful for shared psychosocial stresses (alcoholism, PMS, endometriosis, overweight, or wife abuse).

GETTING A FIX IN OUR OVERMEDICATED SOCIETY

We live in a culture that expects a "quick fix" for everything. We take cold pills to treat our sniffles, diet pills to help lose weight, pills to help us sleep, pain pills for every ache. While medications are often lifesaving and even more often add to the quality of life, we are in many ways a dangerously over-medicated society. Nowhere is that more clear than for midlife women. Millions of people use alcohol and other licit and illicit substances as crutches to get through day-to-day life.

There is a place for tranquilizers. Many people, during a time of great stress, find themselves unable to relax or sleep; the lack of rest in turn makes them less able to cope. Used temporarily in these settings, sedatives, sleeping pills, and tranquilizers have proven valuable. Similarly, in our culture, alcohol serves as a symbol of social relaxation and as something to share with friends.

However, any "substance" as a way of relaxing does not serve as an end in and of itself. Once the immediate effect of the sedative has worn off, the same old problems are still there.

Any woman who finds herself depending on a mind-altering medication has a potential for abusing it. Sedatives and tranquilizers are only a means to an end—temporary relaxation to give a woman more energy to deal with the problems at hand.

Chronic use only depletes your overall energy level. If you find yourself looking toward that "fix" as an end in itself, it's time to get help from a physician or therapist.

When Alcohol Becomes a "Crutch"

Drinking in moderation is an enjoyable pastime for many individuals. Having a drink after work, before dinner, or at other times is a social ritual. Television programs, movies, and books bombard us with the message to "have a drink."

In the Holt-Kahn survey, 5.1% of the respondents said they had more than 2 drinks per day, 22% 1 or 2, and 59% said they have an occasional drink.

Alcohol *may* have beneficial effects. Some physicians advise patients to have one or two drinks each day. Small quantities of alcohol do help some people relax, and may decrease the risk of certain types of heart disease. Unfortunately, many women (and men), don't stop at one or two drinks.

Alcoholism is a democratic disease. Alcoholics come from all walks of life, from bank presidents to domestic workers. Drinking too much isn't a problem associated exclusively with midlife women. "However, there has been an overall increase in the number of women alcoholics in the last 25 years. Whether the increase is a real one, or is accounted for by the fact that women are not as "protected" as before, isn't clear," says Patricia Zak, a recovering midlife alcoholic. "Staying at home, no one saw them except their husbands and families. Some women would sober up late in the day, and even their husbands wouldn't know. Now the ratio of women/men alcoholics may be 50/50."

Women who used to stay at home always had the opportunity to have a few drinks during the day to relieve boredom, change their mood, or "help them cope." Now women who work have opportunities for social drinking at lunch time with business associates and at home in the evenings and on weekends. Women whose husbands came home and unwound with a few martinis now find themselves doing exactly the same thing.

It is difficult to tell when a woman starts to become dependent on alcohol. At first she may use it as a coping mechanism and justify her drinking to herself and others as a means of dealing with her midlife stresses. She may not realize she is an alcoholic.

In the early stage of alcholism, she may be able to compensate at and maintain normal activities, but not for long. Drinking too much can affect a woman's capabilities, especially in the way she thinks and handles problems.

In the middle stage of alcoholism, the addiction begins to interfere with her interpersonal relationships. She may be recognized as a "heavy drinker," or "one who can handle a lot of alcohol." She may begin to have blackouts and hangovers. At this point, she will have difficulty holding her job, because she will find it difficult to get up and go to work. The addictive cycle is firmly established at this time.

In the chronic stage, a woman will have significant difficulty in doing easy, routine tasks, and her reaction time will be very slow. She may have physical problems, including liver disorders. Her brain and heart may be affected. If the alcoholic is not treated at this time, death or "wet brain" (vegetable like existence) will result.

Overcoming alcoholism

Some women consult psychiatrists, psychologists, or clinical social workers about drinking problems. Alcoholism and depression are often linked in cyclic fashion. A mental health counselor will try to understand the relationship between the woman's alcoholism and lifestyle. While talking about the reasons for drinking may be of some use for women in the early stage of alcoholism, of more substantial help for the more advanced drinker is a supportive program on a 24-hour-a-day basis.

Many local hospitals sponsor treatment programs for alcoholism. If you or a friend has a drinking problem, look under "Alcohol" in your telephone directory for the name of a local hospital that treats alcoholism.

Some treatment programs involve staying at the facility for one to three weeks. Programs keep registration lists confidential. People need anonymity to feel comfortable during recovery at their own pace. Some women enter a program in a toxic state. They may also have physiologic manifestations: severe tremors ("the shakes"), disorientation, difficulty in concentrating, unsteadiness, and perhaps delirium tremens (DTs). Within three to five days, the acute withdrawal symptoms will be over.

There is a lot of "cross addiction" between alcohol and certain tranquilizers. This is a deadly combination. If a woman enters an alcoholism treatment program while on tranquilizers, alcohol will be withdrawn first, but she may be supplied with minor tranquilizers for a short time. Gradually she will be helped to withdraw from all tranquilizers. She may begin taking vitamins, particularly B complex and magnesium, because alcoholics usually are low in both. She should also obtain nutritional counseling, because if she has consumed a lot of alcohol and received her calories largely from alcohol, she will have to reeducate herself about healthy eating habits. A good treatment center should have solid medical backup and treat the woman as a "whole person," with a combination of psychiatry and other medical specialities.

The best-known support program for recovering alcoholics is Alcoholics Anonymous. AA is a community of people helping each other. Many women are referred to a local AA group after they complete a several-week treatment center-based program. To locate the nearest AA unit, look in the yellow pages of your telephone directory under "Alcoholics." Many women seek out AA or similar groups in the early stage of alcoholism, before professional help becomes necessary.

Another group, Al-Anon, provides support for relatives of both untreated and recovering alcoholics. Alateen does the same for teenagers with an alcoholic family member.

Prevent complications

Alcohol can alter your body chemistry in ways that affect your menstrual habits, bring on earlier menopause, increase severity of hot flashes, and increase your risk of breast or uterine disease, cardiovascular disease, and diabetes.

Books to read

The Invisible Alcoholic
By Marian Sandmaier
McGraw-Hill
New York, 1980

The Booze Battle
By Ruth Maxwell
Praeger Publishers
New York, 1976

Avoid Becoming a Prescription Junkie

"Popping Valium interferes with learning to deal with stress. These are life changes, and you must adapt to them."

"For women, legal drug and alcohol abuse has become a common hazard that threatens one of every four of us," says Muriel Nellis, author and member of the President's Commission on Mental Health, in her book *The Female Fix* (Boston: Houghton Mifflin, 1980). She refers to drug and alcohol addiction among women as "the unadmitted problem."

Drugs that help you can also harm you, particularly if they are not taken as prescribed. Many women receive prescriptions from physicians for mild tranquilizers or sleeping pills during periods of stress such as illness or the death of a loved one. When women continue taking such pills months—or years—after the stressful event, they may develop an unnecessary dependency. Diet pills and painkillers used routinely also can lead to dependency.

Women have been known to start taking prescription drugs intended for use by another family member. The unused supply in the bathroom cabinet appeals to them at times of stress, and long-term use can result. Often refills are obtained in the original patient's name.

Many women who complain of irritability and tenseness are given prescriptions for the type of drug commonly referred to as anti-anxiety medication. As a mechanism for coping or relaxing, these drugs seem seriously overused and abused.

These tranquilizers are intended to promote relief from anxiety without a feeling of euphoria or drowsiness. One dangerous aspect of these drugs is that their effects are magnified by other drugs and by the state of mind of the user. For example, if you have been drinking alcohol, or are extremely tired, you may receive a double whammy when you take a regular dose of your prescription. Another dangerous aspect is that increasing doses become necessary to give you the same effects, increasing the potential for side effects. And, after taking these drugs in large doses, suddenly stopping can lead to withdrawal symptoms.

"Uppers" include amphetamines, which stimulate the body and create an illusion of energy. In some cases, these pills are prescribed for weight reduction, but there is no evidence that they work over the long run. Also, they may aggravate the cardiovascular system by constricting the small blood vessels, causing mood changes ranging from euphoria to nervousness to irritability.

"Downers" are sedatives. While sleeping pills can be helpful in times of extreme stress (such as before surgery or immediately after the loss of a loved one), they should only be used for short periods. There is a rebound effect from many sleeping pills, and users tend to want to take more instead of getting off them. Also, some sleeping pills cause drowsiness during the day and thus interfere with daytime activities.

Many "prescription junkies" pass into use of illegal substances. In our youth-oriented culture, many women want to be "with it" and try illegal drugs readily available in many communities. Marijuana use has been around at least for 4,000 years. The ancient Chinese learned to use marijuana as an anesthetic in their medicinal preparations. Although marijuana is used today for certain patients—those with glaucoma, as an antinausea agent in cancer patients undergoing chemotherapy, and as a muscle relaxant to control muscle spasms in patients with neurological disease—its mechanism of action is not well understood, and it is still considered a controlled substance.

"Cocaine is an increasing problem among women," says Patricia Zak, a recovering alcoholic who also has a familiarity with the midlife drug scene. "It is appalling to know that 50% of the calls to the 800-COCAINE help line in 1984 were from women. In 1983, men outnumbered women callers three to one. This is frightening, because, at this time, cocaine addiction is the least responsive to treatment."

If you or a friend has become a "prescription junkie," get help. Contact a physician knowledgeable in treatment of addictions. Drug addiction is treated with psychotherapy and education for improved lifestyle. Group therapy seems helpful to many women.

You may also seek help from Narcotics Anonymous (NA). See your local telephone book under "N."

OTHER STRESSFUL FACTORS: CONTEMPORARY FAMILIES

Other major stresses facing many midlife women come from their families. Family life isn't smooth. When problems involve any family member, they almost always also involve good old Mom. As the "strength" of the family, the moms of the world are expected to be everyone else's source of emotional and practical support, often with no one giving them this kind of support in return.

Among the family stresses midlife women face are coping with the midlife changes in the men in their lives; dealing with their grown children and perhaps grandchildren; possibly divorce, widowhood, or remarriage; a new spouses' children and parents, and elderly parents or parents-in-law.

Each woman plays many family roles. She is a daughter, wife, mother, grandmother, mother-in-law, sister. Many women balance these roles along with careers and community interests. The balancing act topples over at times when stresses become too great.

Women today are also in greater decision-making roles than ever before. And many are making decisions to step out of the mold.

"In today's world, there may be three or even *four* generations midlife women deal with—her own, as well as those older and younger," says Jeanne Wielage Smith, Ph.D., Coordinator of the Academic Reentry Program and Instructor, Applied Behaviorial Sciences, University of California at Davis:

> As the prime income-producing generation, midlife women frequently have the prime financial responsibility as well as other supportive roles. As society's traditional care-giver, they have a struggle, and are expected to care for grandchildren and an aging parent. Some assertive women today are saying, "I won't buy into that." This attitude has changed the ways in which some women look at interfamilial responsibilities.

There has been some decrease of the feeling of responsibility. Many midlife women now say, "Let the young parents care for their children. Let the aging parents make their own decisions." Each individual now makes more of his or her own decisions. But this leads to divisiveness. Few would say that family bonds have strengthened in the last 20 years. I think it's been the other way.

Parenting Parents

"Midlife can be a bad time. As soon as our children grow up, our parents become children again."

Most midlife people count having their parents as a blessing. However, when aging parents become incapacitated, mentally or physically, and need a lot of care, psychological tensions can arise.

Many women say they feel "sandwiched in" between caring for children, even after they are grown, and dealing with aging parents. The parents may be hers, or her husband's—or second husband's. Some women feel caught with no one to take care of them and no time to take care of themselves.

Some women have unresolved conflicts with their parents. Once parents become dependent on them, there is little room emotionally to resolve old conflicts. Still, a midlife woman isn't a child and shouldn't feel that she has to "take orders" from a demanding and often irritable aging parent. She can and should assume a more autonomous role.

If you are caught in the "age trap," think about these ideas:

- Be honest with yourself. Acknowledge that you regard the aging parent's requests as unreasonable (if they are).
- Make some adjustments in your routine. For example, acknowledge to yourself that a once-a-week visit might be a more "quality" visit than the twice a week your parent requests. Explain this to your parent.
- If you spend an excessive amount of time with an aging parent, it may be because you feel an unhealthy need to be important to that parent. You may be investing the time out of guilt or to fill the void left by your grown children or by a lack in your marriage.
- If you have difficulty in arriving at a mutually satisfying relationship with your aging parent, consider joining a support group that will help you focus on relieving the stresses women face regarding aging parents.
- Consider engaging the help of a social worker who specializes in geriatrics who will act as a buffer between you and the parent.

The Men in Your Life

"Midlife is a time when couples need a new contract with each other," says Dr. Woloshin. "The contract can be with a husband or a 'significant other.' Recognize that your lives just are not the same as they used to be.

"At midlife, there is a female-male role reversal in terms of psychological needs," says Dr. Woloshin. "Women become more assertive as they age. Men become less assertive and want to be taken care of. They want more nurturing. Couples acknowledging this transition can be accepting of changes in each other."

Other changes in relationships occur because of differences in energy levels. "Many midlife women *do* have more energy than they had when they were younger," says Dr. Woloshin. Women at this stage may have more energy than the men in their lives. When caring for the children is no longer the major focus of a woman's life, she finds that she has new energey for herself and seeks out new activities and interests.

When there are no men in your life

Many women never marry and do not have male companionship. They find that they are complete persons and have productive and happy lives as singles. While the passengers on the ark came in twos, there's no contemporary rule that says you can't sail the ship of life alone.

WIDOWHOOD Becoming a widow is an instant change from being part of a couple to being a single. Most women are not prepared to face the emotional and practical sides of widowhood. They must deal with their own grief, comfort children and other family members, and reorient themselves to new circumstances.

Widows have a major period of realignment of priorities. It takes many women four or five years to work through their loss and readjustment. "They do instrumental things, such as closing of the estate, taking care of investments, routine and mechanical things, although for some these are quite traumatic if they never dealt with the business part of life. After one year, they must establish themselves as single persons," advises Dr. Smith.

DIVORCE Ending a marriage in midlife presents many stresses to the woman who grew up with the notion that marriage was for keeps. After 25 years with the same man, she finds herself single in a world that seems to revolve in couples. She faces new changes and new choices. Her chances include a 5:1 ratio of women to men in her age group. Her choices range from whether to sell her house to where to vacation alone. Financial problems are frequent among divorced women whose energies, put into their husbands' careers and their homes, may *not* be reflected in terms of whose name is on the investments. Potential divorcees need a good lawyer and an assertive attitude to avoid financial woes. However, choices also include establishing herself as a secure, single person, making new relationships and finding new outlets for her energies.

Remarriage and significant relationships

Some women do marry again after widowhood or divorce. Love the second time isn't all moonlight and roses. (As if it were the first time!) Second marriages can work smoothly, but they can also cause unique stresses. When you meet a man at midlife, he comes as a package deal. He may be widowed or divorced, too. The package might include his teenage children, his elderly parents, and other relatives who may or may not accept you. There may be an ex-wife on the scene, or the fond memory of a deceased wife.

How well you are accepted may relate to the circumstances of your courtship. For example, if you were the "other woman" while he was married, the relatives may regard you as a "homewrecker." If you knew him before he was widowed and you marry soon after his wife's death, relatives may think your marriage was too hasty and disrespectful to the deceased. Many midlife women grew up dependent on their families or their husbands. Women's original mindset was "till death do us part." For some divorced women, having to seek a second—or third—husband weighs heavily on their self-esteem.

Some women, after meeting a lovable man who loves them, choose not to marry for a variety of reasons ranging from not wanting to lose substantial alimony payments, to waiting for vesting in a pension plan, to fear of making a mistake.

Many contemporary midlife couples opt for a "living together" arrangement instead of marriage. Women face stresses in relationships with men whether they marry or live together. Many tensions arise over children. In many cases, a woman's own children have grown up and gone away and she marries a man whose teenage children either live with him or visit. She finds herself in a parenting role again. The children may or may not readily accept her. Taube Kaufman, M.S.W., C.S.W., Founder and President, Combined Families Association of America, Inc., offers these suggestions:

- If he doesn't have custody of the children, you may have the children visiting occasionally in your home. Deal realistically with your feelings about the home you and your new love have established. You may feel that the children have no right to be there while their father thinks they have every right to be there. Talk about your feelings with your new husband.

- Don't expect to be able to discipline his children alone. Your role should be to establish with him in advance rules for each child. Post the rules for each child and the consequences for infractions on the refrigerator. Either adult can enforce rules and consequences.
- Remember that you may have to deal with his children's mother at times (his ex-spouse). Keep an open mind and be as friendly and cooperative as possible. Cordial relations between ex-spouses seem to increase enjoyment in remarriage.
- Be aware that jealousies can be evoked in watching the man's relationship with his children. Allow him to have time to relate to his children individually, independent of you.
- Be aware of the ex-spouse's presence (whether alive or dead): Children have feelings about their birth parent. Children don't change their perception of the parent. They remember the parent in the context she was known to them. Encourage children to share their thoughts about the dead or missing parent. Also, allow them the privacy not to share their thoughts, if they don't want to.
- Do not try to be their mother. You never will be. Instead, try to carve out a personal relationship without replacing or displacing their birth mother.

REMARRYING A WIDOWER Remember, in his memory, his first wife remains forever young. He never knew you at the age she was when he courted her. You won't be the first, but second doesn't mean second best. Many second marriages turn out better than the first, even if the first was successful. Some other tips from the Combined Families Association of America, Inc., are:

- Prepare to meet opposition from his children regarding changing his house (if you live in his house). Even if they have grown up and gone away, they will express some opinions on what they regard as their territorial rights.
- If he has been widowed for a long time, he and his children may have developed a very close relationship—closer than they would have been had the first wife lived. The longer the time between her death and his remarriage, the tighter the bond.
- The children may fantasize about how they will take care of Dad in his old age. You interrupt that fantasy. Psychologically, you "knock his daughter off his lap." Children, even grown ones, may never fully forgive you.
- Accept the fact that he may want pictures around the house that include his first wife. There may be a family tree picture, or a pic-

ture that includes his children. If any pictures of her alone, or of the two of them, really offend you, ask that they be taken down. Suggest giving these pictures to the children—or the parents of the deceased wife.

Working

"A lot of ideas regarding menopause are bunk. Scary. I simply went to work full-time and didn't have time to worry about it."

"Women suffer in the workplace because of the myths about menopause. Possibly because some married women exploit the situation. Male bosses judge other women by the way their wives behave, I think."

According to Dr. Smith:

Today's midlife woman expected that her life would be one way and it has often turned out to be another way. Most expected not to be employed, and if they were employed, that their employment would be secondary to marriage and motherhood. They expected to be moving in and out of the labor force. They still do, but only to have children. But the fact that younger women leave the labor force for reasons of motherhood still causes employers to look at all women differently than they regard men, all other things being equal.

Also, there have been changes in the way society and men look at working women. What Betty Friedan did 25 years ago affects 50-year-olds today. The current 25-year-olds are not in harmony with the early concepts of the women's liberation movement. Their lives have been altered, but they don't know what it was like before. The current generation of midlife women is the first generation to reap the benefits as well as dilemmas of the womens' movement. There have been changes in the ways individuals look at each other, and these changes lead to confusion.

Re-entering the working world

Going back to work after years of homemaking is becoming more common each year. In the Holt-Kahn survey group, 80.8% of respondents work, and, of that group, 71.3% work full-time. (This is quite a bit higher than the national average of working women, because our survey group included many professional women.)

Factors that lead a midlife woman back to work or back to school are interwoven. For many, a triggering life event gets them to move on or make a change. The event may be the last child going away to college, divorce or death of the spouse, or a desire to expand personal horizons. Sometimes

these events overlap, and the reasons for reentering school or the w
world aren't clear-cut.

When women decide to go back to school or work, it may be th
time that they have looked at themselves outside of their roles as wive
mothers. They succeed in the personal confrontation and decide
something for themselves. They allow the triggering events to be po
happenings. They recognize that they do have choices, and they r
choices that they will find personally rewarding, either in financial, ca
social, or other areas.

Going back to work isn't an easy matter for many midlife won
"Many women over age 45 often have difficulty with jobs that require a h
level of science and math, because they would have to go back to the be
ning of these fields to catch up," says Dr. Smith, who has counseled many
these women in the course of her work in the Academic Reentry Program a
as Instructor, Applied Behaviorial Sciences, University of California at Dav

> They have a relatively simpler time with arts and humanities, because the
> life experiences are helpful to them.

> Universities aren't necessarily the places to learn new, salable skills. If you
> don't have a skill, go to a spot where you can be trained to do something
> quickly and get paid for it, such as word processing.

> There is a stereotypical attitude that reentering students are mothers who
> are "empty nesters," but that's not true. Most reentering students are in-
> dividuals who are already employed and are looking for new career direction.

> "A colleague, 10 years my senior, maintains that working full-time kept her
> from dwelling on menopause and nearly symptom free."

> "I think menopause has a lot to do with attitudes on life. My boss is 86 years
> old. She has not missed a day's work in 46 years. She looks and acts like she's
> 40. She just remarried. Her philosophy is 'never give in to your illness. It's all
> in your mind.' It worked for her."

Get more than you give: volunteer

One respondent in the Holt-Kahn survey, age 49, married, with four
children and two grandchildren, wrote the following, which nicely
summarizes a fulfulling occupation for many women:

> When you ask if I have worked over the past 25 years, you refer to someone
> who has received a paycheck, I assume. However, I feel you fail to take into
> account those of us who have done community service—also known as
> volunteering. Over the past years I have raised many thousands of dollars for
> various causes in the community. I have been involved in school projects
> when my children were in school.

Today I sit on the Board of Directors of various civic groups in my area. I am a vice president in charge of political and public affairs for Planned Parenthood in my county. I sit on the Family Service Boards for another group, and on the Committee that oversees the budget of various local health and elderly groups. All these activities are performed without pay, but they are as vital and are as much of a time commitment as a job.

Perhaps to the women of the 1980s this is all "small change" and not very important, but to the women of the 1950s, it has been an important part of our lives. Community service should be an area considered and evaluated when you talk about the ways women spend their time.

Plan Now to Be a Nice Old Lady

"I'd like to learn more about understanding emotional feelings—what to do about boredom, fatigue, feeling of loss, some fear of what is to come, and growing old gracefully."

"Enjoy life! We have 30 more years to become involved with our family and any other outside interest we want to pursue. Our minds and our experiences are very valuable assets. We never stop learning. We have a lot to offer the world and we should never lie back and say, 'It's almost over.' A woman's attitude and outlook are what make her a winner or a loser. She has to decide that for herself. Life is what you make it."

What will you make of your life at this point? Are you becoming more accepting of yourself? The oatmeal isn't smooth every day. Some days there are more lumps in it than other days, but it tastes good anyway!

As you look toward aging, plan to become more independent. Even if you are now in an intact relationship, you'll probably live on your own for at least eight years (unless you remarry a younger man). Become more aware of financial matters and operate in as strong and autonomous a manner as possible. "The dependent women will be in trouble. Learn to not be so dependent," counsels Dr. Smith.

As you grow older, learn to separate the stresses you face. Recognize that some stresses are physical, some are practical, and that others are transitory and resolve themselves. Don't let unimportant matters get you down. Be like Scarlet O'Hara who said, "I'll think about that tomorrow."

You may not stop worrying, but you can learn to worry more effectively by categorizing your worries. Once in a while, try making a list of what bothers you. Just as you may try keeping a daily reminder of what you eat so that you can see where to cut out unneeded calories, start a "worry" diary. Separate your worries. For example, don't let your concern about where your husband's elderly father should live interfere with your decision to change jobs. Don't let your daughter's difficulties with her children interfere with having surgery to remove a possibly cancerous mole on your face.

You *can* do something about some of your worries. Take action! Be decisive! Acknowledge that there are some things in life that you just can't do anything about. You're old enough to know that worrying won't help.

Midlife is your time to understand yourself, to love yourself, and to do for yourself.

-

10

"SEX: OVER FIFTY AND STILL NIFTY"

"Menopause certainly has not hurt my interest or ability to enjoy sex with a man I care for. Relax and enjoy this next phase!"

"I'd like to see myths laid to rest. Menopause does not produce dried-up, asexual women."

"What is proper behavior for pre- and post-menopausal singles (recently widowed) who still have a sexual drive?"

"What about the phenomenon of increased sexuality in women over 40?"

"What should I expect in the way of a satisfactory sex life after menopause?"

Today's midlife women discuss sex with other women, with their doctors, and, most importantly, with their husbands and lovers. Many women have emerged from their typecast role of ignorance and passivity about sexual activity.

Many midlife women say they feel sexier than ever. Many find new energy for sexual relationships now that they are no longer tied to worries about becoming pregnant and the day-to-day chores of child rearing. Some men react happily to their newly energized partners. Other men feel threatened by the change. For some couples, this is a time when their sex life stagnates. For other couples, this is an exciting phase of discovery and growth. And for some, failure of one or the other partner to fill sexual needs results in extramarital affairs or marital breakup.

There are many issues regarding sexuality that midlife women share and talk about. These include new sexual freedoms, putting new vitality into a 25-year marriage, maintaining sexual attractiveness in a society that equates youth with sexuality, sex after surgery and illness, losing a partner to another woman (often younger), lack of a partner, and finding new partners.

NEW FREEDOMS: COMMITTED VERSUS CASUAL SEX

Today's midlife woman came of age in a fairly restrictive society. "Nice" girls didn't have intercourse until marriage (or at least didn't talk about it). The worst thing that happened to a married woman was if she or her husband "cheated." Bisexuality and homosexuality were so well closeted that many women didn't know they existed. Women have learned a whole new vocabulary about sexual variances in the last two decades.

Many midlife women have been jolted into the social world of the late 1980s feeling as though they have been in a time warp. *Playboy* and *Cosmopolitan* magazines and X-rated home videos have given them the impression that while they have been content with quick, missionary-style sexual activity while listening for the children, every single has been casually bed-hopping and enjoying widely varied sexual experiences.

Despite the hoopla of the "Sexual Revolution," many people, women and men, have found that physical intimacy connected with a close personal relationship is far more satisfying than casual sex. Even before sexually transmitted diseases became so widespread, many individuals questioned their satisfaction from casual sex.

Women say that having a close friendship with a man before beginning a sexual liaison with him makes the sexual relationship more satisfying. Also, knowing the man well gives her the self-confidence to say no when she doesn't feel the time is right. It can be a delicate balance to be open and spontaneous enough to say yes but self-respecting enough to say no. Striking that balance may be the key to a satisfying sex life.

NEW VITALITY AT MIDLIFE

"Yes, there is sex after menopause!"

"We should have a positive attitude toward a time we can really enjoy. Once in a while a porno video can revive some 'lust' that is foreign to most of us!"

"I have found those who refuse to take medication show personality changes and lack of interest in sex, leading to a weakening of the marital relationship. All of these problems disappear when they turn to medication."—woman gynecologist

Traditionally, we women have let our partners initiate sexual activity. Now men may welcome a show of sexual interest from their partners. "The man may view this as a boost to his sexual self-esteem or a threat to his performance capability," says Domeena Renshaw, M.D., Professor, Department of Psychiatry, and Director, Loyola Sexual Dysfunction Training Clinic, Loyola University of Chicago. She advises frank discussion between partners to prevent anxiety in a man who may be sexually insecure and may misinterpret his mate's changed sexual expression as an excessive demand: "Her renewed interest in sexual activity is an opportunity for both to share and grow in intimacy and capability of enjoyment of sexual pleasure."

Frequency of sexual relations between couples varies. There are no "norms" with which a couple can compare themselves. What suits one couple won't suit another. Some couples are apart geographically because of business travel, and what they miss while away from each other, they "catch up on" when together. Some couples who had intercourse almost every day during the early years of their marriage have made many changes in their sex lives on their way to midlife. Gynecologists say that midlife married women, when asked, report having intercourse on an average of two or three times a week. There are many variations to their habits, however. Some say they don't "get near" their partner when he has a cold, and that two weeks may go by without any sexual activity. Then, on vacation, perhaps in a warm Caribbean setting without any distractions, they may have relations every day, and sometimes even twice a day.

Single women report huge variations in frequency. Some, without a steady dating partner, may not participate in sexual activity for months or years. Those in regular dating patterns may have sexual activity as the "afterglow" of a pleasant evening out once or twice a week. The norms really are so wide and varied that there is no good answer to what is "normal." Satisfaction and needs for satisfaction are individual matters.

ABSTINENCE

"Include details on menopause and sexual desire. We're always assured it's normal and expected to have sex in later life, but I have no interest in it now and feel greatly relieved. Too busy working and doing other things. I think it's probably normal to move on to other things after menopause, though it's great to cuddle anytime. Women should be relieved of guilt about it."

"Deemphasize marriage. Single women are 'women' too!"

Many midlife women are perfectly content without sex. They may be happily single and not miss sex, or happily married to a spouse who for physical or emotional reasons may not want to have intercourse. Some couples find that companionship and nonsexual cuddling fill their physical needs.

Abstinence is a perfectly normal choice. Problems occur only when a couple is mismatched in sexual desires or if a single person is unhappy with abstinence but limited by religious beliefs or lack of a partner.

BENEFITS OF REGULAR SEXUAL ACTIVITY

There are clear-cut benefits to regular sexual activity! Maintaining a constant sex life may help alleviate some menopausal symptoms. In the October 1985 issue of *Archives of Sexual Behavior*, San Francisco State University psychologist Dr. Norma McCoy and physiologist Dr. Julian Davidson reported that women who maintain a consistent sex life are less likely to experience hot flashes. They reported a "close association between increasing irregularity of menstrual cycles, hot flashes, declining estrogen levels and declining frequency of intercourse."

This may happen for several reasons, the researchers said. "The discomfort of hot flashes and other associated symptoms might have an inhibiting effect on sexual behavior. Also, regular sexual activity might have a protective action against lowering hormone levels and therefore its absence is associated with the disruption of cycles." Or, the authors said, "The association between hot flashes and reduced frequency of intercourse may result from some common third variable."

Self-esteem regarding sexual attractiveness wanes for many women because of our culture's equation of youth and beauty. However, with renewed media emphasis on glamour after age 50—and 60—attitudes are changing. You're never too old to enjoy!

Aging can present some specific difficulties, but there are also some specific remedies. In the Holt-Kahn survey, in response to the question "What aspect of menopause concerns your mate the most?" dozens of women replied: "My vaginal dryness." It is a physiological fact that there is reduced lubrication in the vagina after menopause. Many women experience discomfort—even pain and bleeding during intercourse—when the walls of their vagina become thinner and drier. This, however, can be restored by estrogen treatment, saliva, or a vaginal lubricant, such as baby oil, mineral oil, or K-Y jelly.

While some women say there is also reduced intensity of their sexual response, others say it is better than ever. Those who enjoyed satisfying sexual experiences before menopause continue to do so, some with heightened responses because of the absence of fear of pregnancy and lack of interruption by children.

"There are women for whom the risk of pregnancy was a 'turn-on'," says Dr. Renshaw. "For the women who became aroused with the risk, their sense of excitement may be heightened by adding some diversity in sexual activities, such as a shower together, a body-massage, etc."

THE TWENTY-FIFTH ANNIVERSARY DOLDRUMS

"Tell us how to cope with and handle stress. Talk about the importance of 'getaway' trips with your husband."

Often couples have established a "habit" of sex every other Saturday night in the "missionary" position whether they really want to or not. The average frequency of sexual intercourse usually declines with age, and many couples are content to let this gradual slide occur. There is nothing wrong with this, as long as both people are happy. But if you find yourself fantasizing over romantic novels and suspect your husband is doing the same, put a little spice in your life!

Throw a thick, luxurious rug in front of the fireplace and buy a lacy garter belt and a bottle of champagne. Sound hokey? It may be, but it can work. Men often respond to variety, and once the kids are out of the house there is no reason you can't inject some variety into your relationship.

SEXUAL VARIATIONS

The words *fellatio* (stimulation of the penis with the mouth or tongue) and *cunnilingus* (stimulation of a woman's vulva and clitoris with the mouth or tongue) were not part of most women's vocabularies during their high school and college years. Many women admit to having gone to their dictionaries about these words. Some women equated oral sex with "perversions" and considered such acts things that "nice girls didn't do."

"Oral sex is a natural practice carried on in ancient and modern cultures," says Dr. Renshaw. "The lips, mouth, and tongue contain a rich supply of sensory nerve endings. Saliva is an excellent lubrication for intercourse."

Now the prevailing attitude seems to be that any act that the partners consent to and enjoy, which is not injurious to either, is all right. Some individuals may not be "turned on" by oral sex, while others may find it an interesting and satisfying variation. Some find it a gratifying substitute for penile penetration at some or all times because of vaginal discomfort, physical illness, or male impotence.

MASTURBATION

Generations of parents have told their children not to touch their "private parts." Words such as "down there" were used to describe the vaginal areas of little girls. Myths surrounding masturbation were perpetuated. There was the threat that self-stimulation would lead to a range of problems, from insanity to skin diseases.

A real breakthrough in attitudes about masturbation came with the publication of *The Hite Report* (New York: Macmillan, 1976), by Shere Hite. Hite explained that "since almost all women can orgasm easily during masturbation, the well-known difficulty women have in achieving orgasm during sex reflects not a flaw in female anatomy or psychology, but a chauvinist definition of sexuality, reflecting women's second class status in society at large."

"Masturbation is a completely natural form of sexual expression, with exactly the same body responses as happen with intercourse. There is sexual arousal, a sustained arousal plateau, and release by orgasm. The body responds with an increased heart rate, breathing, and muscle tension; these responses may be even higher with masturbation than with intercourse, in which partners must adjust to each other's reactions. The timing (for women as well as men) during masturbation is slightly shorter than intercourse," says Dr. Renshaw. "However, women report that the subjective feeling is different without a penis separating the vaginal walls."

Some sex therapists now use masturbation as an important part of therapy for women who have a difficult time achieving orgasm. With masturbation, a woman can learn how her body functions sexually and better understand her response so that she may then instruct her partner in effective stimulation techniques.

LESBIANISM

There are no real figures on the proportion of women who prefer female sexual partners or may have partners of both sexes, but estimates generally indicate about 10%. Historically, lesbianism was such a taboo subject that it is impossible to estimate whether the rate has increased or remained constant. Now, however, many women are openly acknowledging a preference for female sexual partners.

Many women come to grips with their sexual identities during their middle years. In particular, the current cohort of women in their forties and fifties achieved adulthood during a repressive era, and may have suppressed sexual urges toward other women and become involved in heterosexual relationships, marriage, and childbearing. Some women may have so suppressed same-sex sexual interests that they go throughout life unaware of them; some women become aware of divergent sexual interests at puberty or early adulthood, some at midlife or beyond.

Our culture has become considerably more open about variations in sexual lifestyle over the past two decades. Since lesbian women have often maintained low profiles and monogamous, quiet lifestyles, they have not generally encountered some of the stereotyping and discriminatory practices that gay men have encountered. Some lesbian women have chosen artificial insemination as a means of producing their own children. Others adopt.

SEX THERAPY

In the past 20 years, sex therapy seems to have become an increasingly popular medical specialty. There are sex therapy clinics in most major cities, many connected with universities. "While many mature adults have and can benefit from sex therapy, sex and values are inextricably bound, and no person can change faster or further than their moral values allow," says Dr. Renshaw.

Some psychoanalysts say that many individuals who have sexual dysfunctions need more than sex therapy clinics can offer. Many individuals, whose deeply ingrained attitudes about sex interfere with performance and satisfaction, can be helped by long-term psychotherapy on an individual basis. For many people, a combination of psychotherapy, visits to a sex therapy clinic, and medical attention help.

SEXUAL ACTIVITY AFTER SURGERY OR ILLNESS

> "I'd like to see information on effects of hysterectomy on orgasm."

> "A hysterectomy takes a little adjusting, but is not the end of a satisfactory sex life."

When surgery or illness interrupts a couple's routine of family life, work, play, and lovemaking, the partners have questions about when to resume each activity. Most people ask their doctors about resuming such activities as work, driving, or lifting. But many are reluctant to ask about sexual activity, and many doctors don't bring it up, either. In her book, *Change of Heart: The Bypass Experience* (San Diego: Harcourt Brace Jovanovich, 1985), Nancy Yanes Hoffman included a chapter titled "Sex: The Three-Letter Word Doctors Are Reluctant to Use." She advises that before surgery, ask what you might expect. After surgery, ask what your limitations are, and for how long.

Having some guidelines will make resuming activity easier. After surgery, without some medical advice, the "well" partner has concern about "not hurting" the other, and the postsurgery partner may worry about what is safe.

After Hysterectomy

Hysterectomy is the most frequently occurring major surgery for women. In the Holt-Kahn survey, nearly 30% had experienced hysterectomy. Many women worry about a loss of attractiveness to their mates after this surgery. Hysterectomy, however, should not make a woman any less attractive to her mate.

"All other things being equal, hysterectomy doesn't cause a lack of sexual desire. Just because your uterus and cervix are gone doesn't mean that you won't feel stimulation," explains Dr. Renshaw. "The clitoris is the important arousal center and remains so after hysterectomy, as does the vagina."

A woman facing hysterectomy should ask her physician to draw a simple before-and-after diagram of her insides to show the position of the uterus, cervix, and vagina. She and her mate should look at it to better understand what changes will happen. They should ask how long to plan to refrain from any sort of sexual stimulation and from sexual intercourse after the surgery. In most cases, this length of time is about four to six weeks.

Some women who gain weight after their surgery blame it on the operation, or on their hormone replacement therapy. Sometimes there is four- or five-pound weight gain because of fluid retention due to the hormones, but this can be abated by adjusting the estrogen dosage and cyclic administration of hormones.

Most women will experience little change in their sex lives after hysterectomy, since sexual urges and libido originate from the central nervous system and orgasm is caused by clitoral stimulation. Things may change, however, for some women. Examples follow:

- A woman who identifies sexuality strongly with mothering may feel that sex is "wrong" if not procreative. Ideally, she should seek counseling prior to surgery.
- Women who have had painful intercourse due to fibroids or endometriosis are likely to find a new lease on their sex life, since surgery may eliminate the pain.
- A few women will experience discomfort from scar tissue caused by surgery or radiation. This should be discussed with your doctor, who may recommend more foreplay, stretching with dilators, or vaginal cream to minimize discomfort. Frequent sexual activity and plentiful foreplay will help to elongate and stretch the vagina. The female superior position gives you more control over movement and allows you to avoid painful positions. Many couples use oral sex or mutual masturbation to minimize discomfort.

- After removal of the uterus, the uterine contractions that occur with orgasm are no longer present. This may be a benefit, as these contractions are painful for some women, or this may be experienced as "different."
- In general, a male partner *cannot* tell that a woman has had a hysterectomy unless scar tissue has shortened the vagina.

After Tubal Ligation

Tubal ligation doesn't change a woman's sexual responsiveness in any way. However, the experience of a tubal ligation can unmask underlying sexual problems; couples who experience problems should seek counseling.

After Mastectomy

Resuming sexual activity after mastectomy is a situation thousands of women face each year.

The following problems may affect postmastectomy patients:

- *Fear* After a major life threat, many women lack energy or interest in sexual activity simply because their emotional energy is elsewhere.
- *Negative association of cancer and sexuality* Particularly if a woman's breasts have been a prominent sexual object, she may feel angry, bitter, and betrayed by her body—not a good attitude for loose, uninhibited sexual behavior.
- *Body image change* A woman requires a very strong sexual identity to overcome our cultural obsession with breasts as sexual objects. "She may presume that her appearance also upsets her partner; she may avoid the very closeness that can help heal the emotional pain and stress of surgery," says Dr. Renshaw.
- *Re-defining your partner's role* Often women are worrying about how their partner feels while men are doing the same. Both may hold back from sexual activity because they are afraid the other person will be repulsed or uninterested. Most couples will benefit from discussing these feelings.

Several studies have shown that women who have undergone reconstruction have better self-esteem and body image and dwell less upon their surgery. In part, women with a positive attitude may choose reconstruction. But many people who deal with mastectomy patients say that women with reconstructions come to view the new breast as part of themselves, and certainly being able to dress daily without having to add an external prosthesis must help their self-esteem and, in turn, their sexuality.

Fortunately, the majority of women, both with and without reconstruction, do resume satisfying sex lives, which may even improve as a couple achieves a new closeness from weathering the crisis and as sexuality transcends body changes.

After Cancer

When uterine or cervical cancer is the issue between a couple, sexual activity takes a back seat until there is successful surgical treatment and outcome. "Both partners need warmth and loving support, but may avoid each other at the time when they need each other most. Prolonged petting can help them maintain closeness," says Dr. Renshaw. With mutual sharing and caring, a couple can usually resume sexual relations within a few months after surgery. Each case is different, however, and couples should discuss this question with the gynecologist.

"Some husbands may unconsciously fear that they will contract cancer through intercourse and consequently become selectively impotent. Medical and explicit sexual education can prevent this kind of anxiety," cautions Dr. Renshaw.

After Heart Surgery

In *Change of Heart*,[*] Hoffman says: "Most cardiologists agree that intercourse is no more demanding than climbing two flights of stairs. Most bypassers eventually resume their customary lovemaking without any restrictions at all." Hoffman gives some suggestions for resuming lovemaking after heart surgery that may also interest those recovering from other surgeries/ illnesses:

- Don't eat for at least three hours beforehand. A large amount of blood is redirected to the stomach when you are digesting food, resulting in a decreased amount of blood circulating to other areas of the body. The heart muscle must exert a greater effort to support added physical activity, such as intercourse.

- Begin sexual intercourse when you have plenty of time and are in familiar surroundings; this also reduces the strain on your heart.

---

[*] Excerpts from *Change of Heart*, copyright © 1985 by Nancy Yanes Hoffman. Reprinted by permission of Harcourt Brace Jovanovich, Inc.

Abruptly starting and stopping intercourse can place added strain on your heart.

- Don't consume any alcoholic beverages for at least three hours before sexual activity. Alcohol causes an increase in the heartbeat and makes the heart work harder.
- Try to be comfortably rested. If you are too tired, sexual activity is more draining and more energy-consuming. The best time for exercise, such as intercourse or other forms of physical activity, is after a rest period or in the morning just after awakening.
- Sex is easier when you are content and happy. When you are upset, worrying, or angry, your heart is under strain. These emotional reactions place an additional demand on the heart's work load.

Hoffman discusses positions for intercourse after heart surgery; her suggestions also apply to other postsurgical individuals, not just heart bypassers. She advises exploring through trial and error what modifications in previously used positions are satisfying.

"Remember, sex can't break your Bypass!" Hoffman reminds. But she cautions: "Extramarital sex, sex with someone much younger, or sex with someone new does exert your heart more."

ARTHRITIS

For many with arthritis, the pain may make intercourse difficult or impossible. A gentle hug or caress may bring on discomfort. However, you can direct the caress to a pain-free area and take advantage of good days. The closeness of an embrace may help you feel better. In its *Self-Help Manual for Patients with Arthritis* (Atlanta: The Arthritis Foundation, 1980), the Arthritis Foundation gives some general suggestions regarding sexuality:

- A warm bath or shower prior to sex will be relaxing and soothing.
- A prescribed range of motion exercises will relax your joints.
- Plan to have sexual relations when you generally feel best during the day.
- Time your analgesics so that the effect of the medication will occur during your sexual activity.
- Pace your activities during the day to help you avoid extreme fatigue.
- Experiment with different positions during intercourse and find the ones most comfortable and satisfying to both partners.

The Self-Help Manual includes a short bibliography regarding lovemaking of interest to arthritics and other people with some limitations of movement. Write for information:

Arthritis Foundation
3400 Peachtree Road NE
Atlanta, Georgia 30316

SECOND LOVES

"You may worry that he may have had a better sex life with his former wife than you. She was younger and had a young body. You may be concerned that you can't match up. However, sex may have been the only good thing going for them. You now have a mature relationship based on mutual caring and sharing, in addition to romantic love."

Songs have been written about "the second time around." Recognize that a sexual relationship with a new partner will not be the same as it was with your first. Each partner approaches a new relationship with experiences and preferences individually attained. While you probably shared the enthusiasm of "first love" with your first husband or lover, this aspect may not be present the second (or third) time around. More important, at this time you have the maturity and strength drawn from your past on which to build.

There are advantages in sexual relationships between formerly married or older adults. When your children were young, you may have had trouble finding privacy. If one parent said to the other, "Be quiet, the children might hear you," it may have had a dampening effect on excitement. By the time the children were safely tucked in, the parents were too tired and just went to sleep.

Some say sex with anyone else is not as good as it was the first time around. Age has a lot to do with this attitude. The female may have vaginal lubrication problems and the male may have erection problems. However, the quality of the relationship may make up for the difference.

"In my second marriage, the quality of our relationship superseded sex. The communion between us—devotion, caring, love, understanding—can't be equated to a sexual relationship."

"I'm 56, a widow, and stopped menstruating five years ago. I had a few bothersome menopausal symptoms and haven't taken estrogen replacement because it didn't seem necessary. I hadn't had any sexual experiences until recently. I became involved with a wonderful man, but when our relationship developed to the point of intimacy, I was frightened because my vagina felt

constantly irritated and dry. When I told him about my fear, he was very patient as well as passionate. He touched me as though I was a delicate flower and in such stimulating ways that my old juices began to flow. He eased himself into me as though we had been lovers for years. For other older women faced with this situation: Take your time. You can enjoy if you both understand 'your inner timings'."

LOVING A YOUNGER OR OLDER MAN

Because there are fewer available men in the midlife group than women, single, widowed, and divorced women don't have unlimited choices of partners. Many opt for younger or older men. Many opt for "relationships" rather than marriage.

One midlife widow described her relationship with a younger man as "the honeymoon I never had." She explained that the younger man felt that an older woman would not be as demanding as a younger woman, who might put stress on his sexual performance. An older woman also may give him appreciation in a nurturing kind of way, as well as sexually.

"At any age, a love relationship serves many needs. In addition to sexual satisfaction, a woman needs companionship, caring, and sharing. Many needs can be met without a relationship that depends on an ever-ready erection. There can be kisses and hugs, and sensual touching that leads to sexual fulfillment," comments Dr. Renshaw.

EXTRAMARITAL AFFAIRS

"A man your own age may start looking at younger women. How much will a woman tolerate in extramarital activity?"

"Now, fidelity for a lifetime is almost a myth. Some people are—women are more likely to be faithful than men."

"But I was the one to whom he came back. The others were flings. The others didn't mean to him what I do."

Extramarital affairs have always existed. For midlife women, affairs offer threats as well as comforts on a number of levels:

- *Younger woman* In a youth-worshipping culture, few of us fail to feel a bit bitter at having to compete with younger women who can keep in shape because they have time and money for the health club and aren't flabby from bearing *his* children!
- *Economic security* Unless a woman has had an active full-time career, a marital breakup may mean the difference between a

comfortable lifestyle and a less affluent one. Recent figures by Lenore J. Weitzman in *The Divorce Revolution: The Unexpected Social and Economic Consequences for Women and Children in America* (New York: Free Press, 1985) indicate that the average woman's standard of living declines by 73% with divorce; the average man's increases by 42%. Small wonder women feel threatened.

- *Loss of companionship.*
- *Moral hurt* Even in a liberal society, many women feel that extramarital sex is a sin; or at least unfair.
- *Fear of disease* With sexually transmitted diseases rampant, an extramarital affair can expose an innocent spouse to herpes, gonorrhea, possibly even AIDS.
- The "other woman" often gets a raw deal. You have the family, the social status, the holidays. And even if she successfully breaks up your marriage, she gets a cheater she'll never be able to trust, who (we hope for your benefit) will have to pay child support.
- With patience, you can probably wait it out. One big appeal to affairs is that they can involve commitment-free sex: no bills to pay, no children, no doldrums. But as time goes on, the novelty will wear off and the other woman inevitably will start to demand more time and more money. The homefront will look better and better.

"I divorced my husband many years ago because he was seeing another woman. I'm sorry now. I should have waited it out. I think he would have come back and my life would have been different."

"A change: Women don't divorce as a result of an extramarital affair."

You have to seriously weigh breaking up a marriage over an affair. Since many states have passed "no-fault" divorce laws, there has been a steady decline in women's financial status after a divorce. As our culture has been staggering under the impact of the single-parent family and the feminization of poverty, many people are reevaluating the value of marriage as an economic unit.

Most women coping with the emotional blow of a spouse's affair should consider doing several things:

- Try to get into joint therapy to obtain insight into how to cope and how to strengthen your marriage.
- If he won't get into therapy, *you* go. You can't change him, but you will need all the support and self-esteem you can muster.
- Find a knowledgeable, assertive confidante. Many women, so stunned and upset that they can't think straight, meekly bow out of

a marriage without any demands. You need help mustering your resources and reserves.

- Protect yourself from sexually transmitted diseases. You will be best protected by insisting on condom use and/or a diaphragm and spermicide.

Extramarital Affairs: Bisexual

Once upon a time, all you had to worry about was "other women." It is estimated that about 10% of the adult population prefers same-sex partners at least some of the time, and obviously some of the 10% of men are married, often to women who are shocked and dumbfounded to discover a *male* rival. Here again the same provisos apply:

- Get counseling, either jointly or singly. Women typically blame themselves, which is ridiculous since the dynamics involved often predate your presence.
- Realize you're one of thousands of women this has happened to.
- Don't act hastily.
- Protect yourself from sexually transmitted diseases. Bisexual men are at high risk for AIDS and other diseases.

SEXUALLY TRANSMITTED DISEASES

Sexually transmitted diseases are increasing in epidemic proportions and sometimes are not cured by standard treatments. Gynecologists report dramatic increases in the last 10 years of cases of herpes and other diseases among midlife women.

Women of all ages are concerned. According to the Women's Views Study conducted for *Glamour* magazine in 1985, fear of sexually transmitted diseases was greater than war and peace as a concern to American women. The survey group included women from age 18 to 65. Seventy percent said they were more worried about this issue than they had been the year before.

When midlife women were in school, we learned little about venereal disease (VD) in health class. Historically, VD has been dreaded because of the damage it does to women's and men's sexual systems as well as other parts of the body. Antibiotics developed in the mid-twentieth century cured many forms of these diseases when they were detected and treated in their early stages. However, many strains of disease that once responded to penicillin and other drugs have become more resistant and now are more difficult to treat.

Following is a brief rundown on some common sexually transmitted diseases.

SEXUALLY TRANSMITTED DISEASES (STDs)

DISEASE	FIRST SYMPTOMS USUALLY APPEAR	USUAL SYMPTOMS	TRANSMISSION	DIAGNOSIS	COMPLICATIONS
HERPES SIMPLEX II (Called "herpes") Cause: virus	Variable	Cluster of tender, painful blisters in the genital area. Painful urination. Swollen glands and fever.	Direct contact with blisters or open sores.	Culture taken when the blisters or sores are present.	May be linked with cervical cancer; severe central nervous system damage or death in infants infected during birth.
GONORRHEA (Called "dose," "clap," "drip") Cause: bacteria	2–10 days (up to 30 days)	White or yellow discharge from genitals or anus. Pain on urination or defecation. Possible throat infections. Women may have low abdominal pain, especially after menstrual period. May have no symptoms. Men may have no symptoms.	Direct contact of infected mucous membrane with the urethra, cervix, anus, throat, or eyes.	Women: Culture Men: Culture	Sterility, arthritis, heart enlargement, liver disease, meningitis, blindness. Men: urethral stricture; erection problems.
SYPHILIS (Called "syph," "pox," "bad blood") Cause: spirochete	10–90 days (usually 3 weeks)	1st stage: Painless pimple blister, or sore where germs entered the body; for example, genitals, anus, lips, breast, etc. 2nd stage: Rash or mucous patches (most are highly infectious), spotty hair loss, sore throat, swollen glands. Symptoms may reoccur for up to 2 years.	Direct contact with infectious sores, rashes, or mucous patches.	Blood test or microscopic examination of organisms from sores.	Brain damage, insanity, paralysis, heart disease, death. Also, damage to skin, bones, eyes, teeth, and liver of the fetus and newborn.

(continued)

DISEASE	FIRST SYMPTOMS USUALLY APPEAR	USUAL SYMPTOMS	TRANSMISSION	DIAGNOSIS	COMPLICATIONS
GENITAL WARTS (Called venereal warts, condylomata accuminata) Cause: virus	1–3 months	Local irritation, itching and wartlike growths, usually on the genitals, anus, or throat.	Direct contact with warts	Examination	Highly contagious; can spread enough to block vaginal, rectal, or throat openings.
PUBIC LICE (Called pediculosis pubis, "crabs," "cooties") Cause: 6-legged louse	4–5 weeks	Intense itching, pinhead blood spots on underwear, nits in pubic hair.	Direct contact with infested area or clothes and bedding which contain lice or nits.	Examination	Secondary infections as a result of scratching.
SCABIES (Called "the itch") Cause: itch mite	4–6 weeks	Severe itching at night; raised gray lines on skin where mites burrow, for example, genitals, breast, buttocks, stomach, hands.	Direct contact with infested area or clothes and bedding containing mites.	Examination	Secondary infections as a result of scratching.

DISEASE	FIRST SYMPTOMS USUALLY APPEAR	USUAL SYMPTOMS	TRANSMISSION	DIAGNOSIS	COMPLICATIONS
CHLAMYDIA **Cause: microorganisms**	2 weeks to a month	Women: vaginal itching or discharge; chronic abdominal pain, bleeding between menstrual periods; low-grade fever. May have no symptoms in early stage. Men: Discharge from penis; burning during urination; burning and itching around the opening of the penis. May have no symptoms.	Direct sexual contact.	Laboratory test	
TRICHOMONAS VAGINALIS **(Called "trich," "TV," "vaginitis")** **Cause: protozoa**	1–4 weeks	Women: Heavy, frothy discharge; intense itching, burning and redness of genitals. Men: Slight, clear discharge from genitals and itching after urination. Usually no symptoms.	Direct contact with infectious area.	Pap smear, microscopic identification.	Women: gland infection.

(continued)

DISEASE	FIRST SYMPTOMS USUALLY APPEAR	USUAL SYMPTOMS	TRANSMISSION	DIAGNOSIS	COMPLICATIONS
MONILIAL VAGINITIS (*Called monoliasis, yeast, thrush, candidiasis.*) *Cause: fungus*	Varies	Women: Thick, cheesy discharge and intense itching of genitals; also, skin irritation. Men: Usually no symptoms.	Organisms are present in vagina, rectum, and mouth —usually with no symptoms. Active infection may follow direct contact with infectious person. Also may follow antibiotic therapy.	Microscopic identification	Women: secondary infections by bacteria.
NONSPECIFIC URETHRITIS (*Called NGU, NSU*) *Cause: bacteria or chlamydia*	1–3 weeks	Slight white, yellow, or clear discharge from genitals, often only noticed in the morning. Women: Usually no symptoms. Men: Mild discomfort during urination.	Direct contact with infectious areas.	Smear or culture, usually to rule out gonorrhea.	Women: Pelvic inflammatory disease (PID).

Herpes

Gynecologists say that increasing numbers of midlife women are contracting herpes, often as a result of first-time contacts outside marriage.

The technical name is Herpes simplex or *herpes virus hominus*. For some reason, clinical outbreaks of herpes are more common in women than in men. Herpes outbreaks cause either single or multiple blisters which occur on mucous membranes such as lips or vagina. Herpes simplex I causes most oral "cold sores"; Herpes simplex II, most vaginal herpes. Transmission can occur when a herpes blister comes in contact with any mucus membrane or open cut or sore.

Herpes is most often transmitted through sexual intercourse. It can also be transmitted with mouth-genital contact, or by manual contact during heterosexual or homosexual relations.

You can't always tell if a person has herpes. Rarely an individual can shed the virus even though there are no visible lesions. But more commonly the disease is contagious only if active blisters are present. (A considerate partner will warn his or her lover.)

It takes anywhere between 2 and 12 days from the time of exposure to herpes until blisters develop. Blisters may appear on the mucous membranes around the vagina, cervix, or anus. Sores may last two weeks or more. A person with a first-time bout of herpes may have mild flulike symptoms and a low-grade fever. Bouts of herpes may recur, with sores lasting from a week to 10 days. Sometimes herpes is accompanied by other vaginal infections, such as trichomonas or venereal warts. Urination may become extremely painful. Lymph nodes in the groin may become enlarged.

Herpes can be an extremely debilitating disease. For some, bouts occur when they are under stress, or when they are fatigued or have other illnesses. For most people, however, Herpes simplex virus is a mild nuisance which will gradually get better on its own.

To know whether or not you have herpes, see your doctor and have a culture. It is important that you know whether your lesions are benign or infectious. If you have herpes, you will want to start some treatment to relieve your discomfort. And you'll want to take precautions when you have sexual relations. You don't want to infect your lover. Also, herpes can be transmitted from a woman to her baby at birth, and if you aren't yet out of the baby business, this could be important to you.

Unfortunately, at this time, there is no known cure for herpes.

However, drugs are available through prescription that relieve the pain of the blisters, and, taken prophylactically, may reduce chances of recurring bouts, or lessen the severity of recurrences.

Some physicians prescribe a drug called acyclovir. Oral acyclovir cuts down on the frequency of outbreaks. Acyclovir in ointment form makes blisters heal more quickly and reduces the duration of viral shedding. They also prescribe a topical anesthetic, aspirin, and stronger painkillers. Sometimes a sulfa cream is prescribed to soothe the sores and prevent further infection from other bacteria. Stoxil, an ointment used for herpes in the eyes, offers relief for some women when applied to genital sores. (This should not be used by pregnant women.)

To ease the pain of urination, physicians sometimes prescribe pyridium, an oral medication, which passes through the urinary tract and is excreted in the urine.

Self-help suggestions for herpes

As reported in *How to Stay Out of the Gynecologist's Office* (Culver City, Calif.: Peace Press, 1981), published by the Federation of Feminist Women's Health Centers, some women can avoid recurrences of herpes by taking Vitamin-B complex and Vitamins C, E, and A during times when they are run down or under unusual stress. Other hints about herpes from the Federation's book are:

- Bathe frequently or take sitz baths to keep the sores clean.
- Keep the sores as dry as possible; dry the sores after bathing, perhaps even using a hand-held hair dryer to get rid of any residual moisture.
- Avoid tight-fitting clothing or nylon underwear, which can increase perspiration.
- To alleviate the pain of urine passing over open blisters, the Federation suggests applying petroleum jelly to them before urination. The jelly acts as a seal over the sore, preventing the urine from touching it. If urinations is extremely painful, a woman can sit in a bathtub of lukewarm water to urinate. (Although not always practical, such as when you are at work, this may also be a good idea for avoiding painful urination caused by other infections.)
- Some women apply Vitamin E oil to the sores; others use topical anesthetics, Neosporin ointment, Campho-Phenique, or zinc oxide ointment. Others apply Betadine (povidone-iodine) directly to the blisters.
- The Federation quotes a letter printed in *Prevention* magazine that suggests taking zinc pills orally (50 milligrams of elemental zinc in 348 milligrams of zinc glyconate, once a day).
- The Federation also quotes from a report in the Swiss medical journal *Dermatologica* that suggests that lysine mono-hydrochloride, an amino acid, speeds the healing of herpes.

Lysine can be purchased in health food stores. For more information about this, see:

How to Stay Out of the Gynecologist's Office
The Federation of Feminist Women's Health Centers
Peace Press, Culver City, California, 1981

The Feminist Women's Self-Help Clinic reports learning about several herbal remedies that they say appear to relieve the symptoms of active herpes sores. They say preparations of golden seal, myrrh, ground comfrey root, sap from aloe vera leaves, or peppermint tea bags placed directly on the blisters, have been known to relieve discomfort for some women.

Chlamydia

Since we took school health classes, some other "new" sexually transmitted diseases have become prevalent. One is chlamydia. Although this disease is two or three times more common than gonorrhea, it is not very well known. It affects men and women, but women are less likely to be aware that they have it because they do not feel symptoms in the early stages. Symptoms women may notice include:

- Unusual vaginal discharge.
- Irregular bleeding.
- Bleeding after intercourse.
- Deep pain after and/or during intercourse.

Symptoms men may experience:

- Clear, mucus like discharge from the penis.
- Burning during urination.

Chlamydia is dangerous because untreated symptoms in women can lead to infections in the Fallopian tubes and uterus; this is also known as pelvic inflammatory disease. (See chapter 3.)

Chlamydia is treated with antibiotics. Sexual partners should also be treated to avoid the Ping-Pong effect of reinfection.

Hepatitis B

This is another disease that can be spread by sexual activity. According to a letter to the editor in the September 1985 issue of the *Southern Medical Journal*, some midlife women are bringing back more than straw hats from cruises. The letter indicated that a previously unrecognized group of persons—affluent middle-aged women—may be at high risk of hepatitis B. These women engage in casual sexual activity on board ship, and approximately two months later develop acute hepatitis B. "These cases stress the venereal nature of the disease," said the *Journal*. It went on to warn: "The diverse population aboard many of these ships often includes persons from regions in which the hepatitis B carrier state is endemic. Therefore, vacationers boarding cruise ships should have hepatitis B immunization if they intend to have sexual encounters with new or anonymous partners and they should be aware that they are entering an area with a potentially high prevalence of hepatitis B."

Gonorrhea

The older, more well-known diseases are still with us. Women have fewer symptoms of gonorrhea than men, and it is usually detected later in women than men. Anyone diagnosed with gonorrhea should inform recent partners so that they can obtain treatment; in fact, public health authorities should obtain names of contacts and check to see if they have been treated. In a woman, the gonorrhea germs travel to the uterus, Fallopian tubes, and ovaries. The only symptom she may notice is a white or yellow discharge from her vagina. As the disease advances, she may have some abdominal pain.

Gonorrhea is more difficult to treat in a woman than in a man because the recesses in the woman's tubes and ovaries make the germs less accessible to antibiotics and more likely to survive in spite of treatment. Treatment involves a large dose of penicillin, usually injected, often with follow-up doses of oral tetracycline-type antibiotics, as these penicillin-resistant gonorrhea or concurrent chlamydial infections may not be adequately treated by penicillin. Individuals allergic to penicillin may be given one of the tetracyclines or other antibiotics. Women are usually asked to return for several checkups to be sure that treatment has been effective. Increasing numbers of penicillin-resistant cases of gonorrhea have been reported in recent years.

Gonorrhea, referred to throughout history as the "dose," "clap," or "drip," does not respond to self-help. Complications include pelvic inflammatory disease, joint pains, heart disease, liver disease, meningitis, and blindness. It is important to see your doctor if you think you may have gonorrhea.

Syphilis

Syphilis, like gonorrhea, is usually transmitted through sexual intercourse or oral-genital relations. Although less common than gonorrhea, it is serious because of the complications that occur if the disease is untreated.

Syphilis is usually detected with a blood test. There are three stages in this disease. In stage 1, blisters or sores appear where the germs entered the body, most often on the genitals. This may occur from 10 to 21 days after exposure. Often the sores disappear. However, the disease lurks and will recur as stage 2, when many parts of the body may be infected. There may be a skin rash, fever, sore throat, and inflammation of the eyes. In the final stage of syphilis, the heart, blood vessels, brain, and spinal cord may become involved.

Treatment with penicillin or other antibiotics is usually effective during the early stage of the disease and will prevent complications. It becomes more difficult to treat later on.

Historically, syphilis has been known by many names, including "syph," "pox," and "bad blood."

Other Sexually Transmitted Diseases

There are other, less frequently occurring diseases that may spread through sexual contact. Two examples are pubic lice and genital warts.

Pubic lice

These are tiny bugs ("crab lice," "crabs") that burrow into the skin and suck blood. They thrive on hairy parts of the body, including the pubic mound, the outer lips of the vulva, underarms, the head, and even eyebrows and eyelashes. They cause itching in the area where they have settled. Eggs take from seven to nine days to hatch, and persons infected may notice itching anywhere from one to three weeks after exposure.

Although the most direct way to get pubic lice is through sexual or close physical contact with another person's body, pubic lice *can* be transmitted by sharing linens or bedsheets.

The standard treatment for pubic lice is Kwell, a pesticide sold over the counter in most drugstores. (This is also a standard treatment for head lice.) Shampoo the hairy parts of the body with Kwell to kill the lice. The eggs can be combed out of the hairs, or will fall away by themselves. Contaminated underwear, towels, or bedding should be washed with disinfectant, such as household bleach, in boiling water, then ironed or dried in a hot dryer.

Genital warts

Small bumps on the mucus membrane of the vulva, on the clitoral hood, in the perineum, inside the vagina, or in the anus may be warts. They tend to grow in little cauliflowerlike clusters. They may itch and become irritated. They may be painful during sexual activity and when wearing tight-fitting clothing.

These warts are caused by a virus that is sexually transmitted. Some disappear without any treatment, and some accompany other vaginal infections and clear up when the other infection goes away.

Physicians may remove genital warts with podophyllum, which is highly caustic. They protect the skin around the lesion with an application of petroleum jelly. "In general, it is advisable to use podophyllum only on the outer surfaces of the clitoris and vulva and to wash it off with soap and water between one and four hours after application," advises the Federation of Feminist Women's Health Centers. Be aware that some women have a sensitivity to podophyllum and may have adverse reactions to it. Other medical treatments that physicians use include burning or freezing with liquid nitrogen. Laser has also proven highly effective.

Certain strains of the wart virus have been implicated as a cause of cervical cancer; any women who has warts should be sure to have regular Pap smears. Insist on condom use if your sexual partner has a history of warts.

Other Vaginal Infections

Vaginal infections are among the most common reasons women visit gynecologists' offices, and among the most common reasons for discomfort during sexual intercourse. Some are sexually transmitted, and partners run the risk of reinfecting each other if both do not receive treatment.

Vaginal infections have many similar symptoms, but there are distinguishing characteristics of each. Some can be diagnosed only with specific laboratory tests. Women's self-help groups have instructed women to observe the changes in the odor, color, amount, and consistency of secretions and discharges.

All women have a certain amount of odor from the vulva which, if regular habits of cleanliness are followed, is not unpleasant. Odors resulting from infections have certain characteristics; trichomonas has a strong fish odor, while bacterial infections usually have a fetid odor.

Vaginal discharges help in the diagnosis of infections. Yeast (monilia) usually produces a whitish, curdy, cheesy discharge, sometimes tinged with gray or green. Bacterial infections produce a more creamy discharge. Trichomonas (which may accompany gonorrhea) often produces a greenish-yellow discharge.

With most vaginal infections, the vagina becomes red, swollen, and very tender. The inner labia may also swell and feel sore. There may be intense itching and any friction, such as during sexual intercourse, will be painful.

Trichomonas

This infection, commonly called "trich," is caused by trichomonads, microscopic, parasitic organisms that live in small numbers in the vagina. When their numbers increase, they cause an infection. Trichomonads are usually transmitted during sexual intercourse, *not* by wiping from back to front after a bowel movement. Trichomonads can live under the foreskin of a man's penis or in the urethra, usually without producing any symptoms.

Physicians commonly prescribe a medication known as metronidazole for trichomonas. Taken appropriately, it usually clears up trichomonas within a few weeks. (Be aware that drinking alcohol while taking this drug can intensify unpleasant side effects, ranging from vomiting to diarrhea to a metallic taste in the mouth.) Your partner must be treated simultaneously for the treatment to be effective. A man can also wear a condom during intercourse to avoid reinfection.

Other sulfa-containing preparations are also prescribed in some cases. And, for women who can't take metronidazole, antiseptic douches, such as povidine-iodine, may be helpful, as can meticulous hygiene and soothing baths.

For self-help for "trich," consult the Feminist Women's *Handbook* (see Bibliography).

Yeast (monilia)

While this is not necessarily a sexually transmitted disease, it is included in this section because similar discomforts occur with yeast infections and other infections. However, yeast organisms can live under the foreskin of the penis and be transmitted during sexual intercourse. Yeast infections can also be transmitted through shared towels or bathing suits.

Yeast thrives in a warm, moist environment. Women have the organisms in the vagina at all times. It is only when an overgrowth occurs that the itching and burning sensations result.

Physicians prescribe specific fungicides to treat yeast infections. These may be creams or tablets inserted into the vagina. Before the development of these newer products, gentian violet was used in suppository form or in a liquid for application to the vaginal area. It is still occasionally used, particularly in stubborn cases that do not respond to other treatments.

SELF-HELP. Here's where it's time to take the yogurt out of the refrigerator. According to the Feminist Federation *Handbook*, "The most widely known self-help remedy for yeast conditions is plain yogurt inserted into the vagina. One or two lactobacillus tablets placed in the vagina at the first sign of a yeast condition have the same effects and are generally easier to use."

The Feminist Federation *Handbook* also says that eating yogurt (any flavor) also helps some women bring a yeast infection under control, as does eating quantities of garlic.

Bacterial infections

Vaginal infections that are not caused by trichomonas or yeast may be referred to as "nonspecific vaginitis," "bacterial vaginitis," or "hemophilus" infections. These are often more difficult to treat than those for which specific medications have been developed. Bacterial infections can be transmitted during sexual intercourse. They can also be transmitted by improper wiping after a bowel movement. (Use a front-to-back action with your toilet tissue.)

Physicians usually treat nonspecific vaginal infections with sulfa creams or oral antibiotics after careful diagnosis.

SELF-HELP. An old standby home remedy is a vinegar douche of one or two tablespoons to a quart of water. A douche of 1/2 strength povidone-iodine (Betadine) also may help, says the Feminist Federation *Handbook*. Careful bathing with a mild soap followed by warm, dry air and loose-fitting clothing can help the symptoms of a vaginal infection.

AIDS

AIDS, or acquired immune deficiency syndrome, is the newest and most lethal sexually transmitted disease. The AIDS virus is spread by direct exchange of body fluid, such as blood or semen, or by using contaminated needles for illicit drug use. Fortunately, the virus is not very hardy and does not survive outside the body; hence casual contact through sharing utensils or towels or even kissing has not been shown to transmit the virus. Unfortunately, active AIDS virus is found in semen. The most common form of semen transmission in the U.S. seems to be anal intercourse, during which tears and bleeding from the delicate rectal lining can occur. The vaginal wall is tougher and less prone to tear and bleed, but sperm does travel through the uterus into the abdomen as a result of intercourse. Women who suspect their partners of outside, high-risk sexual contacts, such as promiscuous gay men or prostitutes, should seek the advice of a knowledgeable medical professional about screening for and preventing transmission of the AIDS virus.

Avoiding Sexually Transmitted Diseases

You can reduce your risk of acquiring a sexually transmitted disease. Although some diseases can be passed through other forms of close body contact, sexual intercourse is the commonest route. You won't get these diseases from sitting on a toilet seat. Here's what you can do:

- *Keep your partner to yourself.* Have contact with one person who limits contact to only you.
- *Be selective about your partner.* Be well-acquainted with the person's habits If your partner has contacts with others, you could get an infection without knowing it.
- *Look your partner over.* Ask your partner about any suspicious-looking discharge, sores, or rash. You may be looking at something that is highly infectious.
- *Be clean.* Bathe before and after intercourse. While germs may penetrate the skin before you wash with soap and water, cleanliness can be of value.
- *Have your partner use a condom.* If you have any suspicion about your male partner, ask that he use a condom. It provides good protection against sexually transmitted diseases if put on before any contact and is properly removed afterward.
- *Take care.* Use foam, a diaphragm with spermicides, or sponge spermicides, which kill many infectious agents.
- *Have regular checkups.* If you are sexually active with multiple partners, you should ask your doctor for specific blood tests for some of the sexually transmitted diseases. These tests may not be part of routine examinations.
- *Get simultaneous treatment.* Avoid the "Ping-Pong" effect. If you know you have an infection, tell your partner.Both must be treated at the same time to avoid reinfection.

IS THERE A MALE MENOPAUSE?

"Comment on male menopause. It may be psychological, but it's there."

"What about male menopause and its implications and problems?"

Midlife men are subject to the same basic problem as midlife women. Men worry about losing their good looks, their thinning hair, receding hairline, double chin, paunchy waistline, paying off the last child's college tuition, dealing with aging parents, and the threat of retirement. They share many of the same life stresses as women.

As males age, they also have some hormonal changes that affect their interest in sexual activity. Although some males at midlife are just as sexually active as they were in their twenties, many midlife men experience occasional difficulties getting or maintaining an erection. These difficulties may affect a man's moods, interest in sex, and attitudes about his life and about you.

If you are having midlife sexual doldrums, it may be that indifference has gradually crept up because of your mate's difficulties. While learning to understand your own physiological and emotional changes, learn to recognize situations in him that can lead to further distress. You may be able to help him get help.

Men are different from women (in so many ways!). When a woman has a vaginal problem, she usually calls her gynecologist's office for an appointment. Or she hurries over to the women's health center. Men, on the other hand, often regard a sexual difficulty as a blow to their self-esteem. They may deny they have any problem, or may attribute its cause to some psychological stress, such as tension in the office. Or they may blame the problem on their partner.

To be a helpful, understanding mate, listen to your lover—what he says and doesn't say. If you know him well, you may be able to help him understand the source of his problem. Some male problems *are* "all in the mind." If he is tired, has had too much to drink, or is under extreme stress, sexual interest and capability may be less than usual.

At midlife, the most frequently occurring problems men have that relate to sexual activity are impotence, premature ejaculation, and retarded ejaculation.

There are many different reasons for major male sexual health problems. Some can be helped medically; some require psychological support or help from a sex therapist or psychiatrist. Help your lover recognize when he needs medical help and when you can help him yourself.

Impotence

"Impotence, or the inability to have or maintain an erection, can occur at any age," says Robert Dunbar, M.S.J., health educator and author. In his book *A Doctor Discusses a Man's Sexual Health* (Chicago: Budlong Press, 1976), Dunbar outlines the major forms of impotence:

- Inability to achieve an erection during foreplay
- Loss of erection when the penis is about to penetrate the vagina
- Erection when the penis is fondled by hand or stimulated orally but lost when intercourse begins

- Erection when the man's sexual partner dominates the situation but lost when he is expected to play a dominant role
- Erection when he dominates the situation but is lost when his partner tries to dominate or assume control

Impotence can have physical causes, ranging from hormone deficiencies to diabetes to prostate gland problems. Severe illnesses may cause temporary loss of potency. Drug addiction, excessive use of alcohol, and medications such as tranquilizers and many hypertensive drugs may also contribute to impotence. As men age, they are more likely to develop diseases such as diabetes and high blood pressure. Radiation and chemotherapy can affect hormone secretion and sexual energy. To keep your mate sexually healthy, encourage him to have frequent well-man checkups. Diabetes, if untreated, frequently causes poor erections. High blood pressure may cause decreased sexual potency because of side effects of some antihypertensive medications.

Hormonal imbalance can be discovered by a blood test. In some cases, a deficiency of male hormone can be corrected by administration of male sex hormones, such as testosterone. A poorly functioning thyroid gland may lower the sperm count and also sometimes cause impotence. Appropriate thyroid medication may improve the situation. Male hormones may not be appropriate, however, if the man has certain types of cancer.

Penile splint

"In cases in which a man cannot be helped medically or psychologically, and is unresponsive to treatment or surgical correction, another recourse to make sexual intercourse possible is the penile splint," says Dunbar. "This involves a surgical procedure in which a semi-rigid splint, made of synthetic material such as silicone or polyethylene, is implanted in the shaft of the penis."

While the operation has been successful in many cases, there have been some complications, cautions Dunbar. "In some cases, the splint was fractured during sexual intercourse and had to be replaced. Often the penis will tend to deviate permanently to one side but this has not caused any functional disability. The splint does not provide the same level of satisfaction during intercourse as a normally erect penis, but it is considered a satisfactory alternative to permanent impotence. It will not restore the ability to ejaculate or experience orgasm, however, if these functions have become permanently impaired along with the ability to achieve and maintain an erection."

More recently, an inflatable splint has been developed. "With it, the man can inflate his erection to the desired size at the appropriate time. When finished, the erection is deflated to await reuse," explains Dunbar.

Premature and Retarded Ejaculation

Premature ejaculation is generally defined as the inability of a man to control his ejaculatory reflex. In severe cases, a man will reach orgasm very quickly after he becomes sexually aroused, sometimes even before he penetrates a woman's vagina. Some men ejaculate as soon as they enter. While a man may not be able to hold back his own orgasm as long as it takes his partner to climax, mutual enjoyment will be enhanced if he can sustain his erection.

Retarded ejaculation is not as common as premature ejaculation, but is a problem for many men, particularly those who take certain drugs that interfere with the functioning of the sympathetic nervous system, which controls the sexual response. Tranquilizers, antidepressants, and antihypertensive medications may be contributing factors to retarded ejaculation.

Couples who recognize that their sex life is waning sometimes benefit from techniques they can learn in sex therapy clinics. Trained therapists instruct both partners in ways to enhance enjoyment and overcome male sexual problems. Many midlife men, whose problems have existed for many years, also may benefit from individual therapy with a psychoanalyst.

Prostate Problems

In middle-aged men, a common problem is benign enlargement of the prostate. This can interfere with sexual pleasure as well as urination. The prostate is a small, chestnut shaped gland that surrounds the urethra. The major function of the prostate is to produce the fluid that transports sperm.

Electrosurgical techniques enable surgeons to remove benign overgrowth of prostate tissue, in many cases without an abdominal incision. This type of surgery, when correctly done, does not cause impotence. When properly informed, most patients are not disturbed by retrograde ejaculation (dry ejaculation) which accompanies this type of surgery, because the sensation of ejaculation and orgasm is not altered.

"Recent breakthroughs in surgical techniques have enabled prostatic cancer to be treated without causing impotence. These new surgical techniques make this operation less hazardous than it was years ago," says John E. Garnett, M.D., Northwestern Memorial Hospital, Chicago.

Now that more is known about sexually transmitted diseases, many chronic prostate infections are linked to chlamydia and other infections. After taking a course of antibiotic treatment, a man should return to his physician for a follow-up semen culture to be sure the infection has been conquered. Meanwhile, his partner should also be treated.

Promote Well-Male Health Care

Many women are accustomed to having an annual Pap test and doing breast self-examinations. Some men, however, are less inclined to go to the doctor for routine checkups. Encourage the man in your life to have yearly examinations. Included in the exam will be a prostate examination during which tumors at an early, curable stage can be detected.

A BABY! AT YOUR AGE! (BIRTH CONTROL METHODS)

"I'd like to know how contraception is handled by others during this time."

Age 40 to 55 is a tricky period from the standpoint of birth control. Many couples have tired of worrying about birth control; methods such as the Pill may no longer be safe. Most women suspect they could not get pregnant if they tried, but news of 50-year-old mothers causes a lot of worry. Irregularities in the menstrual cycle, very common at this age, are cause for panic in some women. Dr. Holt estimates that for every 20 women she sees concerned because of missed periods in their forties, 19 of them will not be pregnant. And, unfortunately, sometimes that one has delayed seeking medical attention until she is too far along to have genetic testing performed, or have the option of terminating the pregnancy.

Generally, a woman is considered sterile if she has not had menses for an entire year and is at the expected age for menopause (age 48 to 53). Younger women going through typical symptoms of menopause are probably also safe, but more than one woman going through "premature menopause" in her late thirties or early forties has started menstruating again. Obviously, women who have had hysterectomies are also sterile, as are women who have had tubal ligations (except for the occasional failure). Everyone else needs birth control if she doesn't want a surprise pregnancy.

What are the odds of getting pregnant at 40-plus? A report by Day et al. (*Public Health Report* 73 [1958]: p. 525) found that in 1911 (before widespread availability of birth control) 11% of women 45 to 59 had children under the age of 5; by 1950, 5% of women had children under 5. United States studies have indicated approximately 1 out of 1,000 to 50,000 pregnancies occur in women past 45 (Koren et al., *Obstetrics and Gynecology* 21 [1963]: p. 165). Fertility rates decline gradually for women from the early twenties onward, and more rapidly after age 40. The oldest reported case of pregnancy we could find was age 62 (W. J. Kennedy, *Edinburgh Medical Journal* 27 [1882]: p. 1085). However, the documentation of age in that era is subject to question, and more recent studies with good documentation of maternal age put the maximum age for pregnancy at about 52.

Fertility rates in men also decline gradually after their late teens, but without the dramatic decrease in the forties, and pregnancies have been reported in wives of men in their eighties. However, documentation is even more questionable in male age estimates, since young wives of 80-year-old men have been known to have flings with younger men!

Should you conceive, what are the hazards of childbearing at your age? Probably less than you think! In a report out of Harlem Hospital, in which 90% of the women had less than optimal prenatal care, 94% of mothers over 45 had liveborn infants; 1.2% of the infants had abnormalities (Posner et al., *Obstetrics and Gynecology* 17 [1961]: p. 194). A 1971 series reported 23 healthy infants born to 23 mothers over 45, in a hospital where the majority of women received good prenatal care (Bird and McElin, *Journal of Reproductive Medicine* 6 [1971]: p.48). Basically, with today's availability of good prenatal care, high-risk nurseries, and genetic testing, the chances are overwhelming that your baby will be healthy whatever your age. If you have any serious medical problems, particularly diabetes or high blood pressure, however, risks of pregnancy to both you and your infant are substantially higher.

Miscarriages and genetic abnormalities increase with parental age, and in particular with maternal age. Your personal risks should be discussed in detail with a knowledgeable obstetrician. At age 35, Down's syndrome, the most common age-related defect, is 1/365 births; at age 40 1/109; at age 45 1/32; at age 49 1/12.

The risk of fathers past 40 passing on birth defects is estimated at 3/1000 (*William's Obstetrics* [New York: Appleton-Century-Crofts, 1985]).

Two techniques for screening for genetic defects during pregnancy are available. Genetic amniocentesis, performed at 16 weeks gestation, is highly accurate, with a .5% risk of miscarriage as a result of the test. However, results are not obtained until 20 weeks gestation, requiring a complicated mid-trimester abortion for those couples who choose to abort. A newer technique, chorionic villus sampling, can be performed at 9 or 10 weeks gestation, and results obtained within a few days, allowing for an early abortion; early abortion is a medically safer, faster procedure than is mid-trimester abortion. However, chorionic villus sampling does seem to be associated with a miscarriage rate of 1 to 10%, and is more prone to false positive and false negative readings (missing defects or revealing abnormalities when the baby is actually normal).

Needless to say, deciding on either of these procedures requires careful counseling. But the availability of genetic testing represents a major breakthrough for the woman contemplating a late pregnancy; many women, 20 years ago, unwilling to chance a genetically abnormal infant, either refused to conceive or automatically terminated a pregnancy. Their daughters are now willing to plan infants later in life, due to the availability of genetic screening.

For the vast majority of women in their forties and fifties, however, the burning issue is preventing, not having, babies. For these women, birth control is an important question. Here are the options and the pros and cons of various methods for midlife women.

Sterilization

Surgical sterilization is the single most popular birth control method for couples past 35. *Tubal ligation*, the female sterilization procedure, involves interrupting the Fallopian tubes, which transport sperm to the ovaries and fertilized eggs from the ovaries to the uterus. Since the Fallopian tubes are inside the abdomen, tubal ligation requires surgery performed under anesthesia during which the abdomen is opened with a small incision and either a section of tube is removed, or burned, or a clip or band is placed around the tube. There are a variety of different methods for doing this. One of the most popular, laparoscopic tubal ligation, involves two half-inch incisions and can be done as an outpatient procedure. Women who have had previous abdominal surgery or have certain medical conditions that might make the laparoscopy dangerous may need a "minilap" in which a two-inch incision is made in the abdomen and the tubes are pulled out of the abdomen.

Tubal ligation is very popular, since it has a low complication rate and a low failure rate. A small percentage of women undergoing tubal ligation may require surgery for excessive bleeding. In less than 1% of women, conception will occur after a tubal ligation, but failure rates compare very favorably with those of other birth control methods. A small number of women will have anesthetic complications. One major disadvantage to tubal ligation is that it is permanent, making it inappropriate for women who wish to preserve childbearing potential or for women who have a problem thinking of themselves as "sterile." The risks are small but not nonexistent, and for some women the risks may be higher if they have internal scar tissue or medical conditions that make surgery dangerous (however, many of these women would be far more endangered by a pregnancy!). A few women maintain that a tubal ligation caused heavy menses or pelvic pain, but studies of the rates of these common disorders have not confirmed an increase after tubal ligation.

Vasectomy is the male sterilization procedure. The vas deferens, the tube that transports sperm from the testicles, runs along the surface of the scrotum. It can be pulled out and ligated under local anesthesia. Failures can occur but are not common, and complications such as local infection or bleeding are usually not serious. Overall it is a highly effective, safe procedure. However, many men express concerns over reports that vasectomized male monkeys may have more hardening of the arteries; the role of sperm antibodies reported in men who have had vasectomies is unclear. In addition, some men may feel their masculinity threatened by a vasectomy.

For the couple deciding between vasectomy and tubal ligation, there are several points to consider:

- Vasectomy is safer, since it doesn't require general anesthesia and an intraabdominal procedure.
- No one should be forced into anything.
- Probably the partner who is most adamant about no more children should be the one to take the initiative. That individual should make a decision based on his or her own desires, not pressure from the spouse. Many men have pressured their wives into tubal ligations, only to divorce their wives, who then cannot have children with subsequent husbands.
- A 40-year-old woman is less likely to remarry and want children than a 40-year-old man. Since Mom bears the brunt of pregnancy and child care, she may well be the insistent one.
- Some couples, figuring the wife has done her share with pregnancy and birth control, figure it's the husband's turn to do his part!

Barrier Methods

The old standbys of foam, diaphragms, and condoms are staging a comeback! Health-conscious, educated consumers, who fear the risks of pills and IUDs and wish to control their own bodies, are returning to barrier methods. Studies have indicated that when used as directed, the more effective barrier methods have a failure rate of as little as 2% annually. Barrier methods have several advantages:

- They have virtually no dangerous complications. A small number of women will have allergic reactions to the spermicide or suffer local irritation. Diaphragms may make some women more prone to bladder or vaginal infections. Toxic shock syndrome has been reported in sponge- and diaphragm-users, but is quite rare.
- They may protect against sexually transmitted diseases. Condoms serve as a mechanical barrier to viruses (such as AIDS) contained in semen and shedding from lesions on the penis (venereal warts and herpes can be spread this way). The diaphragm and sponge cover the cervix, and may keep viruses and bacteria out of the uterus. In addition, spermicidal agents in foam, diaphragm gels, and the sponge seem to be toxic to a number of sexually transmitted agents. Using a barrier method does not offer absolute protection against sexually transmitted diseases, but dozens of studies have indicated

that barrier users consistently have lower rates of infection than users of almost any other type of birth control.

Disadvantages of the barrier methods are that some couples find them messy and inconvenient. As a result, some people are prone to "forgetting" to use them, and actual pregnancy rates in couples "in theory" using barriers run from 10 to 20% annually, mostly due to failure to use the barriers! Since many couples during midlife are committed, conscientious users with low potential fertility, barrier methods can be ideal. They are also ideal for the single woman who may have sexual exposure irregularly with different partners, since they are safe and offer protection from disease. For a detailed discussion of the different types of barrier methods, consult a physician or midwife, and read a source such as:

The New Our Bodies, Ourselves
The Boston Women's Health Book Collective
Simon and Schuster, New York, 1984

AMA Guide to WomanCare
Linda H. Holt, M.D., and Melva Weber
Random House, New York, 1984

A New View of a Woman's Body
The Federation of Feminist Women's Health Centers
Simon and Schuster, New York, 1981

Oral Contraceptives

These are mentioned here mainly to warn midlife women against their use. Past the age of 40, particularly for women who smoke, the risk of strokes and heart attacks is substantially increased for oral contraceptive pill users. Very occasionally, a doctor might acquiesce to short-term oral contraceptive pill use in an otherwise low-risk nonsmoker over 40, or might use pills for one or two months to treat a menstrual disorder, but, in general, oral contraceptives should not be used by women over 40.

Intrauterine Devices (IUDs)

IUDs are associated with an increased risk of pelvic infection and heavy bleeding. For these reasons, they have been declining in popularity. One type of IUD in particular, the Dalkon shield, is associated with very serious infections and even deaths. The Dalkon shield was used mainly in the early

1970s, so if you have had an IUD in since then you should seek medical attention and advice about removal. Recently, the manufacturers of the popular "Lippes loop" and the "Copper 7" IUDs took their products off the market, citing legal costs and inadequate profits as the reason. Thus, although IUDs remain popular abroad, the only IUD available in the U.S. (at this time) is the "Progestasert," a progesterone-containing IUD that must be changed annually.

IUDs are *not* for everybody! Since they can increase the risk of infertility, doctors particularly avoid them in women who have not completed their families. Women at high risk for pelvic infections, namely women with previous infections or multiple sexual partners, should generally avoid IUDs. However, for many midlife women, IUDs work well. If you have completed your family and are in a stable, monogamous sexual relationship, you might consider an IUD. Some women who would like to have tubal ligations but are not quite ready to face a surgical procedure or accept permanent infertility choose IUDs instead. Failure rates are approximately 2% annually, and a failure with an IUD in place is likelier to be a tubal pregnancy or result in a miscarriage. An additional problem for midlife women who choose IUDs is that should you be one of the many women who develop prolonged or heavy menses, the IUD is likely to aggravate the bleeding.

Natural Family Planning

The old "rhythm" method that was notorious for its high pregnancy rates has, aided by new knowledge and technologies, given rise to a more sophisticated and reliable form of natural family planning, sometimes called "fertility awareness." The older methods of natural family planning involved figuring out when ovulation normally occurred (usually day 14 of each 28-day cycle) and avoiding intercourse for several days in each direction. But ovulation does not always occur at a predictable time, and most couples going by the calendar sooner or later conceived due to late or early ovulation.

Midlife is a particularly difficult time to use the so-called "calendar" method, since irregular menstrual cycles and erratic bursts of hormone production can result in ovulation at unpredictable times. Temperature charts are not terribly useful for avoiding pregnancy, since body temperature rises *after* ovulation; by the time you realize you ovulated two days ago, you could have already conceived! But new methods for predicting ovulation include cervical mucus changes and chemical tests for hormonal changes that precede ovulation ("ovulation predictor kits"). Many couples are now using fertility awareness successfully for family planning, but you must get careful training in the method before trying it! Local hospitals (particularly Catholic hospitals) and women's centers or your own doctor may be able to direct you to a reputable instructor.

Contraceptive Methods on the Horizon

In many areas of the world, injectable progestins are used for contraception. However, these have not been approved for use in this country for birth control purposes. Injectable progestins are used in the United States on occasion for endometriosis or control of irregular bleeding.

Research is also being done on progesterone-containing implants. Long-acting hormones have the advantage of suppressing ovulation for long periods of time with only periodic effort on the part of the user. They often cause irregular bleeding, and only many years of use by millions of women will reveal whether they compare in safety to other available methods.

Abortion

Virtually everybody condemns abortion as a routine method of birth control. But, at least for now, it remains at times a last resort for the desperate 47-year-old who has had a contraceptive failure or discovers her fetus bears a genetic defect.

If you fear you might be pregnant, seek medical attention quickly, as abortion is safer and simpler during the first three months of pregnancy. It is important not be be scared away from late childbearing by overestimating the risks. But a fact of life is that an unplanned midlife pregnancy can be catastrophic physically, emotionally, and financially for a woman. Many midlife women, realizing the enormous investment of time and energy a child requires, concerned about their own longevity and their responsibilities to the rest of the family, will select abortion.

RESOURCES

Many excellent books are available about sexuality and self-care. Here are a few:

Sex After Sixty
R. Butler and M. Lewis
Harper & Row, New York, 1977.

How To Stay Out of the Gynecologist's Office
Federation of Feminist Women's Health Centers.
Peace Press, Culver City, California, 1981.

A New View of a Woman's Body
Federation of Feminist Women's Health Centers
Simon and Schuster, New York, 1981.

Many newsletters contain information relating to sexuality. You may write to each publisher for details about subscriptions and costs. A few newsletters are listed in the Bibliography.

11

LOOK AHEAD:
THE FUTURE—AND HOW
TO GET BETTER
MEDICAL CARE NOW

Midlife women are in the midst of the second major "public health revolu-tion." Many years ago, the first one involved development of classic public health measures, such as immunizations and purification of water. Our current revolution involves changes in lifestyle and greater individual responsibility for health care. The major unconquered diseases—heart dis-ease, cancer, arthritis, diabetes—will be affected largely by easy-to-change things we can do for ourselves. Our banners read:

> Stop smoking!
> Curb obesity!
> Reduce dietary fat!
> Increase fiber in our diet!
> Exercise more often and more sensibly!
> Avoid overexposure to the sun!
> Drink less alcohol and caffeine!
> Avoid abuse of medications!

In our generation, we have watched the transition from use of doctors' black bags during a house call to computerized diagnostic equip-ment in major medical centers. Now high technology helps doctors detect disease and plan treatment, but the most important weapons in the constant fight for our good health will increasingly come from how we live.

We are indeed the generation with options. In addition to more responsibility for our own health, we now have choices about how and where to be cared for when we do need medical attention. We see more changes ahead in the way we interact with doctors. It is possible to get along better with them! In this chapter you'll learn how.

Also, while taking better care of ourselves, women will become more active in issues relating to health outside the home—opposing environmental pollution and encouraging nuclear disarmament.

HIGH TECHNOLOGY

Women's conversations about health have moved from the sewing circle to high technology. We are the first generation of midlife women to have computers study our bodies, to use electronic banking machines to pay our doctor bills, and to use videorecorders as we exercise to stay fit.

Looking ahead, we see ongoing changes in all phases of our lives. In health care, we are confident that we will continue to benefit from technological changes. Advances since we were girls have affected our health and the health of our children in a myriad of ways. The birth control pill in the 1960s gave us options in contraception and family planning that our mothers never had. Legalization of abortion in the 1970s, although still controversial, gave many women freedom from unwanted pregnancies. Pioneering efforts in organ replacements in the 1970s and 1980s give hope to many individuals with chronic, debilitating, or life-threatening diseases. Vaccines for polio, mumps, measles, and rubella give reassurance against traditional childhood diseases. Methods for genetic testing now help detect dreaded abnormalities in our unborn children or grandchildren.

In the last decade, extraordinary diagnostic equipment has been developed to look inside our bodies. With the help of devices that incorporate computer technology, physicians can see inside us from many angles simultaneously. They can even see a picture of our heart beating on a computer screen!

The future holds many technological possibilities—even in the next decades. For example, "spare parts" will probably become a more significant aspect of care for serious diseases as solutions to the problems of rejection of foreign tissue and transplanted organs are found. Genetic intervention may prevent malformations in future generations. At the same time, genetic engineering can also be used in many ways that may be contrary to the best interests of society. With these advances come ethical, moral, and practical dilemmas we never considered before. Given a limited supply of transplantable organs, who will get organ transplants? Who will give organs? Will genetic engineering always be used for the betterment of humankind? Active, mature women will express their views and help communities decide some of these issues.

BETTER AND LONGER LIVES

With technological advances, we expect better and longer lives. "If we don't destroy ourselves with atmospheric pollution and nuclear weapons, we can expect an accelerated decrease in cigarette smoking and the adverse effects of smoking," says Charles R. Kleeman, M.D., Director Emeritus, Center for Health Enhancement, University of California at Los Angeles Medical Center:

> *Lung cancer now outstrips breast cancer in women as the major cause of death from cancer. This is the direct consequence of the progressive increase in cigarette smoking by women over the last few decades. Women will decrease cigarette smoking with each passing year. That will have a very positive effect on cardiovascular disease and on malignancy. Smoking is the biggest preventable cause of death.*
>
> *Health is predicated on socioeconomic factors. Assuming that our affluence will continue, and that employment will continue at a high level, more people will eat foods high in fiber and more adequate in minerals. The way things are moving in cancer research today, and in our ability to detect cancer, by the year 2000, I expect that cancers due to smoking, high fat intake, and inadequate fiber in the diet will decrease.*
>
> *As individuals, we will do more to prevent cancer than we are doing now. If people gave up smoking, we would eliminate the most common cause of cancer. Reducing our intake of animal fat might reduce gastrointestinal cancer. Removing certain industrial carcinogens would further reduce many cancers.*

Dr. Kleeman also believes that improvements in the quality of life may reach to some very ordinary problems, such as the common cold. "We'll probably have immunization against colds by the year 2000. The common cold is basically a virus infection; we have identified at least seven or eight viruses that cause what we call the common cold. Probably we will have vaccines for colds and use them to immunize the relatively high risk people, as we do now with some flu vaccines," says Dr. Kleeman.

About age: "More people will live to be 100, but not too much beyond that," he says.

MAJOR ISSUES YOU *CAN* DO SOMETHING ABOUT

- *Decrease dietary fat* This may decrease our number 1 killer, cardiovascular disease. In addition, it will probably decrease rates of breast, colon, and prostate cancer.
- *Eliminate cigarette smoke* In our generation, we have moved from widespread smoking anyplace, anytime, to no-smoking sections in

airplanes and restaurants. We have watched a series of alarming messages from the U.S. Surgeon General appear on cigarette packages. We have observed restriction in the ways cigarettes are advertised. The authors suggest another change: *no* smoking!

- *Detect and support early treatment of substance abuse* We have seen alcoholism and pill addiction largely swept out from under the rug. Earlier recognition and acknowledgement of these problems can reduce the costs and catastrophic effects of alcohol, cocaine, and narcotics addiction. These dependencies will be noticed—and cared for appropriately—at earlier stages. More self-help groups with individuals dedicated to supporting each other will lead the way.
- *Encourage more exercise programs in the workplace* In the last decade, the numbers of employee fitness programs has increased dramatically. Employers who include fitness programs as part of the workday believe that these activities help fight overweight, heart disease, and even depressive illness, because people who exercise regularly appear healthier and trimmer, and have a better self-image.
- *Buy fewer products with chemical additives* There are likely to be fewer food additives used in the future, as manufacturers and processors make efforts to assure that only additives thought to be noncarcinogenic and that do not cause adverse effects in our bodies will be used. (When it comes to foods, fresh is best!)

Unfortunately, food additive issues are complicated. Processes that prevent spoilage may involve potentially harmful chemicals. Even "natural" foods can contain traces of naturally occurring toxins or pesticides.

ENVIRONMENTAL ISSUES, FOOD ADDITIVES, POLITICS, AND YOU

While many of today's health problems result from personal health habits—smoking, drinking, abusing drugs, eating too much, not eating the right foods—many of tomorrow's health problems may come from our society itself. You can't solve the dilemma of what to do about environmental toxins by watching what you eat. If the air, drinking water, food sources, and the ground itself have dangerous substances, you as an individual can't stop breathing, drinking, and eating.

That's why there will be more focus on our environment and food additives as health issues in the coming years. We are aware of the adverse health effects of gross radiation exposure and industrial catastrophes such as the ones that occurred in Bhopal, India, in 1985, and at Chernobyl, USSR, in 1986. We are suspicious that more subtle exposures to low-level radiation and toxic waste dumps may cause health problems ranging from hay fever to leukemia. We will look with skepticism at chemicals in our environment and food as technology helps us detect adverse effects. Our challenge will be to eliminate toxic wastes in ways that are safe for us and the environment. Government intervention is probably inevitable, unless individual manufacturers and nuclear plants take on more self-policing responsibility.

Women have traditionally been the guardians of health care and proponents of health issues. While many younger women are now too caught up with their own family responsibilities and beginning careers to become involved in political action programs, now is the time for midlife women to become involved. Of necessity, mature women may have to take a major role in consumer activist organizations relating to our environment and nuclear disarmament.

Health *is* a political issue. Our generation watched the initiation of Medicare and Medicaid during the 1960s, which put our government's hand on our purse strings and made medical costs an issue for taxpayers. Technological advances are expensive and an escalating financial burden to the individual, insurance companies, employers, and the government. Attempts at regulating costs have involved government legislation to encourage prepaid health care services. Even the judicial branch is directly involved in health care; the court's actions in malpractice suits affect physicians' practices. We will probably see increasing government intervention in the form of increasing pressure to keep costs down while maintaining quality of health care.

HOW TO GET ALONG BETTER WITH YOUR DOCTORS

Our survey indicated that, on a one-to-one level, many women are disenchanted with their doctors. Here's what some said:

> *"I've found my doctor to have little time or interest to discuss menopause, and my friends seem to feel the same way about their doctors."*

> *"I hope your tabulation will be an impetus to the medical profession to deal seriously with midlife health questions."*

> *"Even doctors don't understand the frustration of this period of our lives."*

Browsing through the books of the women's health movement shows disenchantment by many women with chauvinistic, inflexible physicians. The book titles say it all: *Male-Practice, Men Who Control Women's Health, The Immaculate Deception, Vaginal Politics, Our Bodies, Ourselves*. How has the image of doctors become so tarnished? And what will a woman do when she realizes that as much as she would like to be in control of her own body, at times she has to rely on a doctor to take care of her?

Feminist literature would have us believe that all gynecologists and surgeons are paternalistic, woman-hating, and mercenary; that's certainly an overstatement of the case. But clearly, there has been a breakdown in communication between midlife women and their physicians.

You can get along better with your doctors if you know a bit more about who gynecologists are, how they are trained, and why they react the way they do; obviously, this description will not fit all gynecologists. However, with this information, you may have more successful interactions with your doctor—or at least a better idea about why you should find another doctor!

Why Doctors Are That Way

Realize that medical students—male and female—are not selected for warmth, empathy, and humanism. Although medical school admissions officers may give lip service to humanitarian qualities in applicants, most classes are filled with students who have stellar academic records. Often they obtain straight-A grades by "grinding" through a rigorous undergraduate science curriculum, not by developing social skills.

Once in medical school, academic survival depends on being able to memorize huge quantities of material, usually by cutting off all involvement with friends, family, and outside interests. Then, four more years of gynecologic and/or surgical training require grueling hours and many sleepless nights. Most doctors who survive training do so based on grim determination and raw stamina, again often at a great cost to their personal lives.

After the just-described 12 or more years of "tunnel vision," during which few normal human contacts are maintained, it is not surprising that some gynecologists and surgeons come across as abrupt and unsympathetic, especially considering their hectic schedules. It is indeed remarkable that despite the fact that nurturant, humanistic qualities are neither sought after nor rewarded during training, a fair number of gynecologists and surgeons are actually warm, caring individuals.

Doctors have been trained to identify and treat disease. Surgeons in particular see their role as identifying and removing disease. Meanwhile, you, as a patient, want a sympathetic ear, and safe, effective, and easy cures. Frequently these goals mesh nicely. You go to the doctor with an ear infection, you get an antibiotic, and you are soon cured. Unfortunately, much frustration results when these goals do not come together so neatly.

An example: Mary M. has chronic pelvic pain. Her doctor runs a lot of uncomfortable tests, the results of which are normal. He concludes there is "nothing wrong." She goes to another doctor, who runs the same set of tests again. He cannot identify the source of her pain, but recommends a hysterectomy because, after all, he is trained as a surgeon, and if she is having pain in her female parts, why not take them out?

A third doctor notes that she has been "doctor shopping," tells her it is "all in her head," and suggests she see a psychiatrist. Mary M. is still in pain, but she is also frustrated and has spent a lot of money.

Sound extreme? This routine happens all too frequently. The problem is that the doctors see their role as being either identifying or "ruling out" known diseases, while Mary M. sees their job as alleviating her pain, preferably without major surgery. Neither side is completely right. Doctors have a tendency to say "there is nothing wrong with you" when what they really mean is that "using currently available tests, I cannot identify any known disease that explains your problem." Patients, used to miracle cures, do not always accept that the same medical profession that can do heart-lung transplants cannot cure an arthritis pain. Unfortunally, doctors are not miracle workers; they are simply human beings working with a limited set of tools.

There is no easy answer to this gap between expectations and reality. Doctors can help by simply being honest and admitting that they are stumped, if they are. Most women can probably accept that a doctor may not be able to find the source of the problem, but understandably resent feeling brushed off or ignored.

As a health care consumer, you can help by doing your homework, learning as much as you can about your body, and being realistic in your expectations from your doctor. And both sides will benefit from simple courtesy. Patients are frequently incredibly nasty to a doctor's office staff but are upset when treated in kind. Also remember that receptionists and nurses are human beings, too, and respond to simple courtesies.

Female Versus Male Doctors

"My doctor(male) has been very unsympathetic and noncommunicative during this period of my life. I would like to see a chapter with advice on how to cope with this. The more secrets we get out of the closet about this the better!"

"Do you have any data on differences, if any, in quality of information and care between female and male gynecologists: pro-surgery or anti-surgery, or types of medications suggested?"

"I found male M.D.s very unhelpful. I would recommend a female M.D. for women every time."

"I always thought how nice it would be if I had a woman gynecologist. Now I have one and she is just as abrupt and quick to leave the room after the examination as the male doctors. She doesn't sit still long enough for me to ask my questions. I end up talking to the nurse."

Until very recently most doctors were male. Only in recent years have large numbers of women doctors been available. Many women attribute negative qualities to their doctor's sex. Perhaps once women have free access to doctors of both sexes they will discover that it is the individual, not the sex, that is critical. Many women who have gone through medical training have done so by "out-machoing" their male classmates. Medical training requires many traditionally "feminine" qualities such as empathy and nurturance, as well as many traditionally "male" qualities such as aggressiveness and perseverence. Don't make sex-linked assumptions about doctors. Instead, seek the personal characteristics that are important to you in a physician.

What Motivates Doctors?

"I thought these would be the relaxed years of my life, but the problems and painful part has offset the enjoyment! The doctors have been no help at all. They're as uninformed as I am. All they know is how to charge money!"

In a "fee-for-service" system, doctors make money for performing services. Much has been written about the economic motivation of physicians in this system to maximize their income by performing expensive, well-remunerated surgical procedures rather than practicing preventive medicine. Probably most doctors do not consciously recommend procedures and surgery to make money, but the incentive under a fee-for-service system is certainly toward a definite, lucrative procedure, such as a hysterectomy (which can generate a $500 to $2,000 fee for a morning's work) instead of spending many office hours listening to a woman complain about her heavy periods and trying alternative therapies.

As a health care consumer, you can avoid this possible bias by obtaining a second opinion from someone with no economic interest in surgery (and no ties of loyalty to the first doctor) or by joining a prepaid health care plan, in which doctors do not benefit from the number of surgical procedures they do. However, in a prepaid plan, critics say there may be an incentive to undertreat rather than to overtreat. (More about prepaid plans later in this chapter.) At this point, you may feel you can't win; however, if you see a variety of doctors, you may get a feeling for a reasonable "middle ground" approach.

"Do No Harm," Said Hippocrates . . . Malpractice

Doctors view the basic problem of malpractice as being greedy lawyers and patients who expect perfect results. Trial lawyers and injured patients see the problem as incompetent doctors. The truth probably lies somewhere in between. But, there is no doubt that unless malpractice premiums level off and doctors lose their fear of lawsuits, medical costs for "defensive medicine" tests will continue to rise rapidly.

Doctors will increasingly band into large groups to pool costs. They will start to avoid certain types of patients and procedures considered "high risk." Doctors will probably increasingly tend to practice "cookbook" medicine and conduct every imaginable test, and be loath to use their intuition or an original approach, since extensive testing and traditional treatment are "safer"—less likely to result in a lawsuit in the event of a bad result. The doctor-patient relationship will no doubt suffer, as the constant threat of litigation can make doctors touchy and defensive—not exactly a good mindset for relaxed, empathetic care.

COMPETITION: ALTERNATIVE FORMS OF HEALTH CARE DELIVERY

"When I moved to Sacramento, I had trouble getting a recommendation about new doctors. Everyone I asked was in an HMO, and their doctors don't see people who aren't in their HMO."

"I didn't want to join the HMO at work because I like my gynecologist, who has his own office. I had a hard enough time finding him. Once I found him I've stayed with him for years. Why do I like him? Once I lost a Tampax inside of me. When I went to him to have it retrieved, he didn't laugh."

"I never got anything from my health insurance company except a bill. Now I get newsletters and free health education classes. That's the effect of competition."

We can now shop for health care the way we shop for the houses we live in and the cars we drive. We can compare prices and quality. We look for covenience and good service. In the last two decades, competition between health care providers, insurance plans, physicians, and hospitals has forced these providers to become more efficient in the way they do business—and in some cases, to reduce costs.

Once health insurance on the job was considered a "fringe" benefit. Now we expect health insurance, and we expect options. Some employees have as many as half a dozen or more health care benefits options: a traditional indemnity-type policy, a major medical policy, or coverage by one of several types of prepaid plans such as Health Maintenance Organizations (HMOs) or Preferred Provider Organizations (PPOs).

HMOs and PPOs are known as "alternative" forms of health care delivery because they offer an alternative to the system of paying a doctor a fee for each service (fee-for-service system) and then waiting for reimbursement for some or all of the charges by an insurance plan.

It's nice to have options, but making the choice can be confusing. Here are a few guidelines about some alternatives.

What's an HMO?

Harold S. Luft, in *Health Maintenance Organizations, Dimensions of Performance* (New York: Wiley Inter Science Series, 1981), explained that the central feature of the HMO concept is a contract between you and the HMO whereby for a fixed annual fee the HMO agrees to provide a stated range of comprehensive health care services. "The intent is to change some of the financial incentives in the medical care system. Under the usual fee-for-service system, the provider's income is directly related to the number of services rendered. With a fixed payment per enrollee, the HMO's net income is inversely related to the number of services provided, and there is a financial incentive to reduce the number of unnecessary procedures. HMOs also have an incentive to provide appropriate preventive services in order to avoid larger expenditures in the future. Thus the HMO theoretically emphasizes health maintenance, rather than simply sickness care."

There are two basic types of HMOs:

1. The group practice or staff model that hires or contracts with a limited number of doctors in one or more health care centers
2. The individual practice association (IPA) that contracts with a large number of individual doctors who operate out of their own neighborhood offices

What's a PPO?

There are many varieties of PPO arrangements, but, in general, an employer or insurance company contracts with a group of doctors to provide a stated range of services. In a PPO, doctors are paid on a discounted fee-for-service basis. Consumers are not restricted in their choice of physicians, but they are given financial incentives to use the preferred providers participating in the PPO arrangement.

"Blue Cross is involved in setting up PPOs as well as HMOs. We see both as part of an overall technique in capping health care costs. The PPO is appealing to many people who don't want to opt for the HMO concept," says Richard Allen, Marketing Director, Empire Blue Cross/Blue Shield HMO in New York. Consumers have a wider choice of physicians in a PPO than in an HMO.

There has been a rapid increase of enrollment in alternative health care plans for many reasons. Some people have found appeal in the idea that for a fixed prepaid fee, they can budget for all of their health care needs, both in the doctors' offices as well as in the hospital, and be assured of quality of care. For some, the convenience of having access to many specialists is the big draw. For others, the lack of claim forms is appealing.

In 1986, according to InterStudy, a nonprofit research, education, and consulting organization whose mission is to improve the performance of the U.S. health care system by stimulating competition and market forces, more than 21 million people belonged to nearly 500 HMOs. By 1995, over half of the U.S. population will be enrolled in price-competitive health plans, such as HMOs, predicts InterStudy.

By 1990, according to InterStudy, an estimated 57.4 million Americans, will belong to prepaid health plans, as opposed to individuals covered by traditional indemnity health insurance.

Typical of many of the now approximately 300 rapidly growing HMOs across the country is the Empire Blue Cross/Blue Shield HMO in New York, which in early 1986 had more than 55,000 members. Services provided on a prepaid basis range from well-baby checkups to open heart surgery. "If our medical group doesn't have the resources, we obtain the services elsewhere. For example, when a bone marrow transplant was needed, we discovered the medical facility with the highest success rate with this procedure in Seattle; our HMO covered the patient's procedure there," says Richard Allen. He continues, "On a more everyday level, our plan and others are growing because of our comprehensive coverage. For example, there's no limit to the number of visits a member makes to a doctor. If a women needs many followup visits to her gynecologist after starting on estrogen replacement therapy, that's all covered."

If you have the option of joining a "Federally qualified" HMO, you will have a chance once a year to reevaluate your choice. According to the HMO Act of 1973, the Federal law under which HMOs operate, HMOs must offer reenrollment periods each year, and a chance to change plans. People faced with alternatives in health benefits may switch from an indemnity insurance plan to an alternative type, or vice versa.

"The fact that the numbers of Americans in HMOs increases each year, indicates a degree of satisfaction," says Timothy Bell, a nationwide consultant to the health care industry, based in Reston, Virginia.

HMOs also have built-in quality checks. Plans must comply with Federal and state regulations. Plans have "peer review" systems to monitor care given by individual doctors and precertification routines before surgeries.

Choosing a Health Insurance Plan

When faced with the choice of health care options, make an informed choice. Read all the literature you receive about the plans available to you. Once no one read the fine print on their health insurance contract until they were sick! Once you only had to seek a doctor whose skills you trusted and whose style you liked. That was back in the days of no choice. Now it's different. You have options.

Today's medical marketplace is complicated. You have to consider the whole picture, often choosing a plan that will meet your needs ranging from sniffles to organ transplants! Most of us are unprepared for this kind of medical marketplace. To help you get through the maze, following are some important questions to consider.

Costs

- What are the monthly fees? How much will you pay? If you are employed, how much will your employer pay toward the plan?
- What will you have to pay for out-of-pocket costs? HMOs and PPOs often cover practically all medical costs for services provided *at their facilities and by their doctors*. Traditional insurers, while giving more choice of facilities and doctors, may or may not cover "routine" office visits, or may have a deductible (amount you pay before coverage starts) or a "copayment" (fraction of the cost that you pay).
- What will be your total costs—either if you are healthy or have an illness? Your costs will be the sum of:
  Monthly fees +
  Deductibles +
  Copayments +
  Medications (some plans cover prescription drugs) +
  Use of any doctors or facilities not covered by the plan
- For fee-for-service doctors: What are their charges for a first visit? Subsequent visits?

Quality

- Can you inspect a list of the doctors' credentials? Are they Board certified or Board eligible in their specialties?
- Is the doctor or medical group respected in the community?
- Is the office clean and appealing? The office staff efficient, courteous, and helpful?
- Is the hospital they use well-respected?

Convenience and availability

- Are the plan's doctors' offices convenient for you?
- Do they have hours that fit your schedule?
- Is there adequate weekend and nighttime availability?

Private, "solo practitioner" doctors are more likely to be personally available to you on weekends and evenings. However, large groups and "systems" like HMOs usually have a well-organized "call" system, assuring that someone will be available at all times. There are advantages and disadvantages of each. Some women feel strongly about having "their" doctor available, and might fare better with a solo practitioner (but are in trouble when he/she is on vacation or too exhausted to think straight). Other women simply want some readily available source of advice and care, and may feel more comfortable calling an "on-call" doctor with a question. As one woman who had just joined an HMO said: "I always felt awful calling our pediatrician when my baby was sick, knowing how busy and tired he always seemed. It is nice to be able to call someone for advice who you know isn't 'on' seven days a week!"

- Are the hospitals the doctor/group uses convenient?
- Can you get appointments quickly for urgent and routine care?
- How long do people wait in the office once they get there for an appointment?

Miscellaneous but very important issues to ponder before changing your health care plan

- Do you have a relationship with doctors you like? Can you continue seeing them or would you have to change to other doctors if you change plans? Or, if you have no contacts with physicians, do you know how to go about locating physicians when you need them?
- Do you have a "preexisting" condition? If you have any illness *before* joining a new plan, it may not be covered! Insurers try to avoid what they call "adverse selection," meaning that sicker people who join their plan will cost a fortune and drive up their costs. You could be in trouble if you switch plans to have surgery, for example, and the new insurer refuses to pay for care for your fibroids since they were a preexisting condition.
- What will happen if you want care not covered by the insurer? In many cases, you are out of luck. Areas such as mental health, treatment for substance abuse, cosmetic surgery, or experimental procedures may not be well covered. An HMO or PPO may not cover care if you are not treated at their designated facility, so if you are used to making an annual trip to the Mayo Clinic, be sure you're covered!
- "Federally qualified" HMOs are required to offer a wide range of covered benefits; compare these with the benefits offered by tradi-

tional health insurance plans. While HMOs may limit your choices regarding facilities, traditional insurance may limit your choices by requiring large deductibles and copayments.

Special concerns for single women or any woman who might become single (that's all of us!)

Women often are underinsured for health care. They may be part-time employees, self-employed, or have employers who are not required to offer health insurance. Some women are dependent on their husband's health insurance policy, and find themselves with no coverage after divorce or widowhood. Laws regarding dropping of an ex-spouse or widow from insurance plans are changing. Now, under some plans, a woman can continue in the plan by paying for her own coverage.

If you are contemplating divorce, think about your health care insurance, and if you lack adequate coverage on your own, negotiate for your husband to continue you on his policy, if possible. Or be sure that you can get a comparable arrangement on your own. Also, be sure to consider the needs of minor children. They must be insured on at least one parental or school policy.

IT'S A SMALL WORLD, AFTER ALL

In summing up the progress relating to women that began during the United Nations' "Decade for Women" (1975–1985), Dr. Halfdan Mahler, Director-General of the World Health Organization, could have been addressing American midlife women when he said:

> There is now more discussion of women's problems, more advocacy of their rights, more understanding of their position. There is also a new awareness by women themselves.

> The special role of women in health care is often taken for granted. The health care system depends on women. Yet the paradox is that, while society depends so heavily on women to provide health care, women's own health needs are often neglected. Women themselves are often unaware of the nature and extent of the problems.

> Changes in family structure, values and roles often increase women's burdens. While there is no inherent conflict in the many roles women are expected to play, their task is not always appreciated and valued by society at large, and the support needed from family and society is not always forthcoming.

Clearly, more attention must be given to women's health and the part they play in health and development. There are still wider considerations—employment, education, social status, the freedom to plan their families, equitable access to economic resources and political power. We cannot view health in isolation from these.
(Reprinted with permission from World Health, *April 1985.)*

It's a new you out there. It's a new world. Keep your bones strong. Drink milk. Be active to stay fit and flexible. Eat enough fiber in your diet and cut down on fats. Drink less alcohol. Don't abuse medications. Stop smoking. Keep your head on straight. Be nifty—long after 50. Look ahead!

GLOSSARY

ADRENAL GLAND. A triangular-shaped gland attached to the top of each kidney that secretes various substances that influence every body system.

AIDS (acquired immune deficiency syndrome). A sexually transmitted disease triggered by a virus that destroys the body's immune system.

AMENORRHEA. The absence of menstrual periods.

ANDROGENS. A group of hormones that promote the growth and development of muscles, hair, and bones. Generally referred to as "male" hormones.

ATHEROSCLEROSIS. Hardening of the arteries.

ATROPHIC VAGINITIS. Thinning of the vaginal walls, which may result in susceptibility to infections and discomfort during sexual intercourse. This results from low estrogen levels following menopause.

AUGMENTATION MAMMOPLASTY. A plastic and reconstructive surgical procedure in which the breasts are enlarged.

BAND-AID STERILIZATION. *See* TUBAL LIGATION.

BARTHOLIN'S GLANDS. Small glands on the side of the vaginal opening that secrete lubricating fluid; they become more active during sexual excitement.

BASAL CELL CARCINOMA. A type of skin cancer. Basal cell carcinomas usually occur on individuals who have been exposed to sunlight for long periods of time. They are slow-growing and can be surgically cured when removed completely.

BENIGN. Not cancerous.

BETADINE (povidone-iodine). An iodine-based antibacterial soap that is sold without prescription; it is used as a douche for vaginal bacterial infections or trichomonas, in conjunction with other medications.

BIOPSY. Removal of a small amount of tissue or fluid from the body for diagnostic examination.

BISEXUAL. A person who may select a sexual partner of either sex.

BREAKTHROUGH BLEEDING (BTB). Vaginal bleeding that occurs between menstrual periods. Some women have BTB during the first 2 or 3 cycles after starting oral contraceptives; spotting is BTB with less blood loss.

CALCITONIN. A hormone secreted by the thyroid gland that inhibits the release of calcium from bone.

CARCINOMA IN SITU. Localized cancer that has not spread to underlying tissues.

CERVICITIS. Inflammation or irritation of the cervix.

CERVIX. The lower part of the uterus that extends into the vagina.

CHEMOTHERAPY. Treatment of a disease by chemicals, usually used in reference to cancer treatment.

CHLAMYDIA. A common sexually transmitted disease that can cause vaginal discharge, pelvic inflammatory disease, and infertility.

CHOLESTEROL. A substance found in animal fats, blood, and nerve tissue. High cholesterol levels in the blood may lead to atherosclerosis, or hardening of the arteries.

CLIMACTERIC. The gradual transition from reproductive years of regular ovulation to the postmenopausal years when the ovaries cease functioning. This spans the ages between the late thirties and mid fifties.

CLITORIS. The female organ that includes the small protrusion above the vagina. This is the primary female organ of sexual arousal.

COITUS. Specifically describes the sexual act with the penis in the vagina.

CONDOM. A sheath of rubber or animal skin placed on the penis prior to coitus that catches seminal fluid and prevents sperm from entering the vagina. Condoms also act as barriers to bacteria and help prevent passing of infections between partners. Condoms are sometimes referred to as "rubbers."

CURETTE. A metal instrument that looks like a cutout spoon used to scrape the lining of the uterus; used in a D and C.

CYST. Benign sac or pocket within a tissue or organ that fills with fluid or semisoft material. Cysts can occur in breasts or ovaries.

CYSTIC BREASTS. Breasts in which many or frequent cysts or cystic growths occur.

CYSTITIS. Urinary tract infection. Technically, the word means inflammation of the bladder.

D and C (dilatation and curettage). A common operation in which the cervix is stretched (dilated) and the lining of the uterus is scraped with an instrument called a curette.

DIAPHRAGM. A rubber dome on a flexible rim that covers the cervix and fits behind the pubic bone; used for birth control. Use of a diaphragm also requires use of about a tablespoonful of spermicidal cream or jelly.

DIETARY FIBER. The plant materials that are resistant to the action of the digestive enzymes of the human small intestines. Important for preventing constipation and may reduce the risk of colon cancer as well.

DIURETIC. A medication, food, liquid, or other substance that causes an increase in the amount and frequency of urination; often used in high blood pressure medications or to relieve bloating.

DOUCHE. Introduction of a stream of water or other solution into the vagina to help treat vaginal infections; not an effective method of birth control.

DYSMENORRHEA.   Painful menstruation, often accompanied by cramps.

DYSPAREUNIA.   Painful sexual intercourse.

ENDOCRINE SYSTEM.   Includes thyroid, adrenal glands, and pituitary gland, plus ovaries in women and testes in men; ductless glands that secrete hormones and other substances that affect other organs of the body.

ENDOMETRIOSIS.   A condition in which uterine tissue is found in other nearby parts of the body, such as the ovaries or Fallopian tubes or around the bladder or rectum. Endometriosis sometimes causes irregular and painful menstruation, pain during coitus, or infertility.

ENDOMETRIUM.   The uterine lining tissue.

ESTROGEN REPLACEMENT THERAPY.   Treatment in which estrogen or a combination of estrogen and progestin is taken to relieve symptoms caused by the lack of estrogen produced by the body.

ESTROGENS.   A group of hormones that, in women, are produced in the ovaries and trigger ovulation and stimulate growth of the lining of the uterus. They are also produced in other tissues, such as body fat; they are responsible for development of secondary sex characteristics. Men also have lower levels of estrogens made mainly by conversion of male hormones.

ETHINYL ESTRADIOL.   A synthetic form of the ovarian hormone estrogen.

FACE LIFT.   This is the common term for plastic surgery procedures known as meloplasty and rhytidectomy. The plastic surgeon usually will make an incision running from the temple down the front of the ear and up the back of the ear into the scalp. The skin of the face and neck is then released from the underlying tissue. A variety of different approaches are then used. Some surgeons will pull up the heavy tissue underneath the skin before the skin itself is pulled up. Other plastic surgeons tighten the muscles of the neck and remove the fat from the neck. These procedures may be done separately or in combination. The older type of face lift in which only the skin is moved upward and the excess removed has been replaced by these newer methods.

FIBROIDS.   Fibrous, noncancerous growths, most commonly found in or on the uterus.

FSH (follicle-stimulating hormone). A hormone secreted by the pituitary gland that stimulates production of ovarian hormones and prepares the ovary for ovulation.

GENITAL WARTS. Also called venereal warts, these are small, rough bumps on, in, or near the genitals; caused by a virus that is transmitted through direct contact.

GYNECOMASTIA. An extreme form of enlarged breasts. Can be corrected by plastic and reconstructive surgery. *See also* MACROMASTIA.

GONORRHEA. A sexually transmitted disease caused by specific bacteria; transmitted by direct contact. Also referred to as "the clap." It requires treatment with antibiotics and must be reported to public health authorities.

GnRH (gonadotropin-releasing hormone). The hormone made by the hypothalamus that stimulates the pituitary gland to produce gonadotropins.

HERPES SIMPLEX. A sexually transmitted viral disease that causes the skin to erupt in recurring blisters, commonly on the genitals and mouth; can be spread when herpes blisters come into contact with mucous membranes, an open sore, or a cut. A related virus, herpes zoster, causes chicken pox and shingles.

HORMONE. Substances produced in organs, glands, or tissues that are carried in the blood to distant parts of the body to stimulate specific activity or production of other hormones. These naturally occurring substances affect every part of the body and are affected by many factors, including stress, exercise, and nutrition.

HOT FLASHES. Sensations of heat in the skin that occur when estrogen levels are low; also called hot flushes.

HRT. Hormone replacement therapy. *See* ESTROGEN REPLACEMENT THERAPY.

HYPERTENSION. High blood pressure.

HYPOTHALAMUS. A coordinating center of the brain located just above the pituitary gland.

HYSTERECTOMY.   Surgical removal of the uterus.

IATROGENIC.   Caused by a physician.

IDIOPATHIC.   Occurring without known cause.

INCONTINENCE.   Uncontrollable urination or defecation.

IUD (intrauterine device).   A birth control device consisting of plastic or other material inserted into the uterus. An IUD usually prevents a fertilized egg from implanting on the uterine wall.

KEGEL EXERCISES.   A set of exercises which involve tightening the vaginal/urethral muscle called the pubococcygeus muscle. Used to increase bladder control and sexual pleasure.

LACTOBACILLUS ACIDOPHILUS.   Bacteria found in yogurt and other milk products; also found in the vagina and the intestines, where it keeps down the growth of yeast. Suggested by some women to decrease yeast overgrowth in the vagina. Can be inserted into the vagina in the form of plain yogurt, as a douche, or as a tablet.

LESBIAN.   A woman who prefers to have sexual relationships with women.

LH (luteinizing hormone).   The pituitary hormone that stimulates release of the egg from the follicle and formation of the corpus luteum.

LIBIDO.   A term used by Sigmund Freud that now means sexual desire or sex drive.

LIPECTOMY.   A plastic and reconstructive surgical procedure to remove fat.

LIPOPROTEINS.   Proteins combined with fatty substances (lipids) in blood plasma. Increased levels of high-density lipoproteins (HDL) in the blood are associated with a reduced risk of cardiovascular disease. Excessive amounts of low-density lipoproteins (LDL) increase an individual's risk of cardiovascular disease.

LUMPECTOMY.   Surgical removal of a breast tumor and sometimes other breast tissue without removing the entire breast.

MACROMASTIA. This refers to large breasts; if severe, it is called gigantomastia. Women complain of back and neck pain, breast pain, and difficulty in breathing. This can be corrected with plastic and reconstructive surgery.

MALIGNANT. Designating an abnormal growth that tends to spread and may be threatening to health and life.

MAMMOPLASTY. Plastic surgery on the breast.

MAMMOGRAPHY. A method of photographing the breast by using X rays; the procedure is intended to reveal or confirm breast lumps.

MASTECTOMY. Removal of a breast.

MASTURBATION. Stimulation of one's own body, particularly the genitals, to produce sexual pleasure and orgasm.

MENARCHE. The first menstrual period.

MENOPAUSE. Cessation of menstrual periods; defined as the passage of an entire year without menses in absence of any pathologic state which has caused that cessation.

MENORRHAGIA. Excessive menstrual bleeding.

MESTRANOL. A synthetic estrogen.

METABOLISM. General term that designates all chemical changes occurring in food nutrients after they have been absorbed from the gastrointestinal tract; also designates the cellular activity involved in using these nutrients.

NEUROTRANSMITTERS. Chemical compounds that relay impulses among neurons and enable nerve cells to communicate with each other. Examples are serotonin, norepinephrine, and dopamine.

NONSPECIFIC URETHRITIS. A common condition in which symptoms of a bladder infection (urinary frequency, urgency, and pain) occur in absence of an identifiable urinary tract infection.

NORETHINDRONE. A synthetic form of the female hormone progesterone.

OOPHORECTOMY. Surgical removal of one or both ovaries.

ORGASM. The climax of sexual activity in which tension causes muscle contractions that force out accumulated blood from erect and engorged genital tissues. In males, orgasm culminates with ejaculation. In females, it causes rhythmic contractions of uterus and vaginal tissues.

OSTEOCLAST. A cell that assists in the resorption of bone by the body.

OSTEOMALACIA. Softening of the bone due to loss of calcium.

OSTEOPOROSIS. Bone loss resulting in weak bones. A disease characterized by a decrease in bone mass and an increase in porosity and fragility of the bones. It occurs more quickly after menopause, when estrogen levels are low.

OVARIES. Two endocrine glands about the size of unshelled almonds; located on either side of the pelvic cavity near the opening of the Fallopian tubes. Ovaries produce hormones: estrogens, progestogens, and androgens. They release ripe eggs during a woman's reproductive years.

OVULATION. The release of an egg from an ovary.

PAP SMEAR. A screening procedure to detect cancer of the cervix; samples of cells from the cervix are smeared on a microscope slide for examination; recommended for all midlife women once a year.

PELVIC INFLAMMATORY DISEASE. An infection of the reproductive tract that can lead to infertility. It is commonly caused by *Neisseria gonorrhoeae*, which causes gonorrhea, but other organisms may also be involved.

PITUITARY GLAND. An endocrine gland about the size of a kidney bean; located at the base of the brain. Responsible for producing a wide variety of hormones, particularly FSH and LH.

PLASTIC SURGERY. Surgery done with appearance in mind; can involve either reshaping normal structures or repairing injuries or destruction of tissue due to disease. Also referred to as cosmetic surgery or reconstructive surgery.

POLYPS. Soft red growths with stems that commonly occur in the uterus and rectum. Polyps usually are noncancerous, but can bleed when irritated.

POSTMENOPAUSAL. Pertaining to the period of a woman's life after cessation of the menses.

PREMATURE MENOPAUSE. Menopause that occurs before the normal time (i.e., age 40), often due to surgical removal of the ovaries.

PREMENSTRUAL SYNDROME (PMS). A combination of physical and emotional symptoms occurring one to two weeks prior to menstruation. The symptoms of PMS include breast tenderness, swelling, headache, acne, depression, and moodiness.

PROGESTERONE. A hormone that, in women, is produced in the ovaries and prepares the lining of the uterus during the second half of the menstrual cycle to nourish a fertilized egg.

PROGESTIN. A synthetic hormone, similar to the hormone progesterone.

PROGESTOGENS. Steroid hormones that include progesterone and other hormones that have similar effects.

PUBOCOCCYGEAL (PC) MUSCLE. A band of muscles surrounding the vagina, urethra, and rectum that can be contracted voluntarily; the muscle contracts involuntarily during orgasm. Kegel exercises involve tightening this muscle (the PC muscle).

RECONSTRUCTIVE SURGERY. Surgery that attempts to "reconstruct" parts of the body ravaged by injury or disease; often used to refer to breast reconstruction after mastectomy.

RHYTIDOPLASTY. Cosmetic surgery procedure intended to reduce appearance of facial wrinkles.

SPECULUM. An instrument that is inserted into a body opening to look inside. A vaginal speculum is used to see the vagina and cervix.

SPOTTING. *See* Breakthough Bleeding.

STRESS INCONTINENCE. Inability to hold urine during laughing, coughing, sneezing, or running.

SUBCUTANEOUS MASTECTOMY.   A technique used by surgeons in which the breast is removed but the overlying skin and nipple are not removed. The technique is often used in precancerous conditions. Reconstruction can be done using a silicone prosthesis.

TESTOSTERONE.   The strongest of the male hormones, made by the testes; also produced in small quantities by females either by the ovary or by conversion from estrogens in skin and fatty tissue.

THERMOGRAPHY.   A technique to detect the presence of cysts and cancers by measuring temperature differences between tissues. Generally not as accurate as mammography.

TRANSILLUMINATION.   A diagnostic technique to confirm the presence and size of breast lumps that involves shining a strong light through the breast.

TRICHOMONIASIS.   A sexually transmitted disease caused by parasitic protozoa (*Trichomonas*) that live in the vaginal tissue; the major symptom is a yellowish or greenish odorous discharge.

TUBAL LIGATION.   Closure of the Fallopian tubes done by laparascopy; this involves tiny incisions that can be covered by Band-Aids. Also known as Band-Aid sterilization.

UNOPPOSED ESTROGEN.   Estrogen treatment without the sequential treatment with progestin.

VAGINITIS.   Inflammation of the vagina, usually marked by discharge, itchiness, and pain. Any vaginal infection is a form of vaginitis. It is called "nonspecific" when several types of bacteria are present, or when the type of bactaria cannot be identified.

YEAST.   Also called *Monilia* or *Candida Albicans*, this is a fungus always present in the vagina and rectum, but when overgrown, causes infection and discomfort. The major symptom may be a cheesy vaginal discharge.

BIBLIOGRAPHY

Menopause

Budoff, Penny Wise, M.D., *No More Hot Flashes and Other Good News*, Warner Books, New York, 1984

Buchsbaum, Herbert J., ed., *The Menopause*, Springer-Verlag, New York, 1983

Cutler, Winnifred Berg, Ph.D., Garcia, Celso-Ramon, M.D., and Edwards, David A., Ph.D., *Menopause, a Guide for Women and the Men Who Love Them*, W. W. Norton & Co., New York, 1983

Gray, Madeline, *The Changing Years*, New American Library, New York, 1981

Greenwood, Sadja, M.D., *Menopause Naturally*, Volcano Press, San Francisco, 1984

Reitz, Rosetta, *Menopause, a Positive Approach*, Penguin Books, New York, 1983

Utian, Wulf H., M.D., *Menopause in Modern Perspective*, Appleton-Century Crofts, New York, 1980

Health in general

The Boston Women's Health Book Collective, *The New Our Bodies, Ourselves*, Simon and Schuster, New York, 1984

Duncan, G., M.D., ed., *Over 55: A Handbook on Health*, The Franklin Institute Press, Hillsdale, N.J., 1982

Federation of Feminist Women's Health Centers, *A New View of a Woman's Body*, Simon and Schuster, New York, 1981

Federation of Feminist Women's Health Centers, *How to Stay Out of the Gynecologist's Office*, Peace Press, Culver City, Calif., 1981

Gordon, Michael, *M.D., Old Enough to Feel Better: A Medical Guide for Seniors*, Chilton Book Co., Radnor, Penn., 1981

Holt, Linda Hughey, M.D., and Weber, Melva, *The American Medical Association Book of WomanCare*, Random House, New York, 1982

Scully, Diane, *Men Who Control Women's Health*, Houghton Mifflin, Boston, 1980

Herbal therapies and other alternatives

Parvati, Jeannine, *Hygieia*, Freestone Publishing Co., Berkeley, Calif., 1983

Fitness

Berland, Theodore, *Fitness for Life, Exercise for People Over 50*, Scott, Foresman & Co., Glenview, Ill., 1985

Fonda, Jane, *Women Coming of Age*, Simon and Schuster, New York, 1984

Higdon, Hal, *Fitness After 40*, World Publications, Mountain View, Calif., 1977

Marshall, John L., M.D., *The Sports Doctor's Fitness Book for Women*, Delacorte Press, New York, 1981

Hysterectomy

Morgan, Susanne, *Coping with a Hysterectomy*, The Dial Press, New York, 1982

Nugent, Nancy, *Hysterectomy*, Doubleday and Co., Garden City, New York, 1976

Premenstrual syndrome

Harrison, M., *Self-Help for Pre-Menstrual Syndrome*, Matrix Press, Cambridge, Mass., 1985

Lark, S., *Pre-Menstrual Syndrome, Self-Help Book*, Forman Publishing Inc., Los Angeles, 1984

Witt, R., PMS—*What Every Woman Should Know About Pre-Menstrual Syndrome*, Stein & Day, New York, 1983

Osteoporosis

Notelovitz, M., et al., M.D., *Stand Tall: The Informed Women's Guide to Preventing Osteoporosis*, Triad Publishing Company, Gainesville, Florida, 1982

Miscellaneous special concerns

American Medical Association, *Straight Talk, Non-Nonsense Guide to Better Sleep*, Random House, New York, 1984

Arthritis Foundation, *Self-Help Manual for Patients with Arthritis*, Arthritis Foundation, Atlanta, Ga., 1980

Bing, Elisabeth, and Coleman, L., *Having a Baby After Thirty*, Bantam, New York, 1980

de Beauvoir, Simone, *The Second Sex*, Alfred A. Knopf, New York, 1953

Friedan, Betty, *The Feminine Mystique*, Dell, New York, 1977

Greer, Germaine, *Sex and Destiny*, Harper & Row, New York, 1984

Hoffman, Nancy Yanes, *Change of Heart: the Bypass Experience*, Harcourt Brace Jovanovich, San Diego, 1985

Kahn, Ada P., M.P.H., "Help Yourself to Health" series: *Arthritis, Diabetes, Headaches, High Blood Pressure*, Contemporary Books, Inc., Chicago, 1983

Weitzman, Lenore J., *The Divorce Revolution: The Unexpected Social and Economic Consequences for Women and Children in America*, The Free Press, New York, 1985

Nutrition

Bailey, Covert, *The Fit or Fat Target Diet*, Houghton Mifflin Company, Boston, 1984

Brody, Jane, *Jane Brody's Nutrition Book*, Bantam Books, New York, 1982

Orbach, Susie, *Fat Is a Feminist Issue*, Berkeley Publishing Co., New York, 1978

Roth, Geneen, *Feeding the Hungry Heart*, The Bobbs-Merrill Company, Indianapolis, 1982

Sex and sexual health

Butler, R., and Lewis, M., *Sex After Sixty*, Harper and Row, New York, 1977

Dunbar, Robert, *A Doctor Looks at Male Sexual Health*, Budlong Press, Chicago, 1976

Hite, Shere, *The Hite Report*, Macmillan, New York, 1976

Lumiere, Richard, M.D., and Cook, Stephanie, *Healthy Sex and Keeping It That Way, A Complete Guide to Sexual Infections*, Simon and Schuster, New York, 1983

Westheimer, Dr. Ruth, *Dr. Ruth's Guide to Good Sex*, Warner Books, New York, 1983

Drug abuse and alcoholism

Maxwell, Ruth, *The Booze Battle*, Praeger Publishers, New York, 1976

Nellis, Muriel, *The Female Fix*, Houghton Mifflin, Boston, 1980

Sandmaier, Marian, *The Invisible Alcoholic*, McGraw-Hill, New York, 1980

Newsletters

A Friend Indeed is a newsletter published 10 times a year as a resource, support, and forum for menopausal women. For information, write to:

> Editor
> A Friend Indeed
> 4180 Wilson Avenue
> Montreal PQ., H4A 2T9
> Canada

Better Health Newsletter, a quarterly publication written and edited by physician-writer Dorothy Young Riess, M.D., is dedicated to better health through education; each issue includes a special article on women's health. For a free copy and subscription information, write to:

> Dorothy Young Riess, M.D.
> 2750 W. Washington Blvd, No. 270
> Pasadena, Calif. 91107

The Melpomene Report, published three times a year, is the journal of the Melpomene Institute for Women's Health Research, which serves physically active women and girls. The journal reports on research on the effects of exercise on women throughout the lifespan, including ongoing studies of osteoporosis, pregnancy, nutritional needs of athletes, exercise patterns of runners, athletic amenorrhea, and physical activity for older women.

For information on the cost of subscriptions, as well as individual issues, write to:

Melpomene Institute for Women's Health Research
2125 East Hennepin Avenue
Minneapolis, MN 55413

National Women's Health Report is a bimonthly digest of current information on health issues concerning women of all ages and lifestyles. Preventive medicine and health maintenance are key themes. For information or subscription, write to:

Editor
National Women's Health Report
P.O. Box 25307
Georgetown Station
Washington, D.C. 20007

Nutrition Action, published 10 times a year, contains practical information including time-saving, health-enhancing recipes and tips; it is published by the Center for Science in the Public Interest, a nonprofit consumer advocacy group concerned with achieving better health through better nutrition for all Americans. For information on subscription and a free flyer listing all of CSPI's publications, write to:

Nutrition Action
Center for Science in the Public Interest
1501 Sixteenth Street, N.W.
Washington, DC 20036

PMZ newsletter, an update to *Menopause, Naturally*, quarterly, includes comments and ideas from readers who have found ways to increase their zest and their contributions to the world in the second half of life. For information, write to:

Sadja Greenwood, M.D.
201 Edgewood Avenue
San Francisco, Calif. 94117

Sex Over Forty, a newsletter directed to the sexual concerns of the mature adult, monthly. For information, write to:

> Saul H. Rosenthal, M.D.
> Sex Over Forty
> P.O. Box 1600
> Chapel Hill, N.C. 27515

APPENDIX

Since few numbers on how women really experience menopause were available, we decided to gather some on our own. We needed cohorts of women in the midlife years. We decided to mail questionnaires to several cohorts, including high school and college classmates of co-author Ada P. Kahn, since we could obtain mailing lists for these groups. We used high school class lists, for the early 1950s, from several Chicago high schools, including Roosevelt High School, and from one California high school. Additionally, women in the Northwestern University classes of 1955 and 1956 received mailings. Another source was Women in Communications, Inc. (formerly known as Theta Sigma Phi), into which co-author Kahn was initiated as a student, a little more than 30 years ago. Questionnaires were also given to many colleagues and acquaintances in the 45-60 age range.

A final group surveyed was women gynecologists in the 40-60 age group who are Fellows of the American College of Obstetrics and Gynecology. This is a fairly select group, since at the time they attended medical school very few women became physicians, and in particular, few women pursued surgical specialties such as gynecology. We felt that this was an important group to survey, even though there were only 126 women gynecologists in this age group (identified by the ACOG listing of Fellows). We thought that this knowledgeable group of women ought to have good insight into the issues we wanted to discuss. We were expecting a mere handful of replies from this busy group (94 percent of the doctors who replied are in full-time practice), but to our surprise we received 52 replies (a 41 percent return rate), which we thought was impressive for an unsolicited, mailed questionnaire.

Overall, we mailed 2,000 questionnaires and received back 967. We were happily astounded! We had expected a 10 percent return rate. What was even more impressive is the time many women took to write lengthy comments. We have included many of these comments in the text, hoping that you will find them as interesting as we did.

The numerical results of the questionnaire follow each question: both the number of replies and the percentages (in parentheses) are given.

1. Your age now: Median age was 51, with 60% of the women between 50 and 55 and 94% between 45 and 60.

2. Do you still have regular periods? 762 replies

No:	670	(70.6%)
Yes:	279	(29.4%)

3. Marital status: 962 replies

Married:	700	(72.6%)
Single:	92	(9.6%)
Widowed:	45	(4.7%)
Divorced:	124	(12.9%)

4. Number of children: 950 replies

0:	138	(14.4%)
1:	78	(8.2%)
2:	304	(31.4%)
3:	271	(28.0%)
4:	130	(13.4%)
5:	21	(2.2%)
6:	4	(0.4%)
7:	5	(0.5%)
(Average:	2.3)	

5. Number of grandchildren: 913 replies

None:	713	(73.7%)
1:	90	(9.3%)
2:	58	(6.0%)
3 or more:	52	(5.6%)

6. Do you have high blood pressure? 961 replies

Yes:	132	(13.7%)
No:	829	(86.3%)

7. Do you have diabetes? 945 replies

Yes:	13	(1.4%)
No:	932	(98.6%)

8. Do you have heart disease? 942 replies

Yes:	21	(2.2%)
No:	921	(97.7%)

9. Have you experienced hot flashes? 949 replies

Not at all:	348	(36.7%)
Mild:	449	(47.3%)
Severe:	152	(16.0%)

10. Has vaginal dryness been a problem? 953 replies

Not at all:	598	(62.7%)
Mild:	315	(33.1%)
Severe:	40	(4.2%)

11. Has loss of urine with coughing, laughing, or jogging been a problem? 959 replies

Not at all:	494	(51.5%)
Mild:	315	(43.8%)
Severe:	45	(4.7%)

12. Has excessive weight gain been a problem during the last few years? 959 replies

Not at all:	405	(42.2%)
Mild:	446	(46.5%)
Severe:	108	(11.3%)

13. Has depression been a problem during the last few years? 956 replies

Not at all:	513	(53.7%)
Mild:	381	(39.9%)
Severe:	62	(6.5%)

14. Have you ever had a mammogram? 966 replies

No:	363	(37.6%)
Yes:	603	(62.4%)

15. Have you had a hysterectomy? 817 replies

No:	574	(70.3%)
Yes:	243	(29.7%)

16. Do you have your ovaries? 933 replies

No:	125	(13.4%)
Yes:	805	(86.3%)
Don't know:	3	(0.3%)

17. How often do you see a doctor? 939 replies

Annually:	405	(43.1%)
Biannually:	171	(18.2%)
As needed:	376	(37.4%)

18. Do you take vitamins? 938 replies

No:	351	(37.4%)
Yes:	586	(62.5%)

19. Is osteoporosis a concern to you? 955 replies

No:	234	(24.5%)
Yes:	721	(75.4%)

20. Do you take calcium supplements: 949 replies

No:	382	(39.5%)
Yes:	565	(59.5%)

21. Did your doctor prescribe calcium supplements for you? 647 replies

No:	439	(67.9%)
Yes:	208	(32.1%)

22. Are you using any kind of hormone? 956 replies

No:	701	(73.3%)
Yes:	255	(26.7%)

      Breakdown of hormones taken:

Estrogen cream:	28	(2.9%)
Estrogen pills:	118	(12.2%)
Progesterone:	22	(2.3%)
Est./Prog. pills:	91	(9.4%)
Male hormones:	3	(0.3%)

      (Numbers here do not add up exactly since a few women reported using more than one form of hormone.)

23. Do you drink alcoholic beverages? 955 replies

None:	127	(13.3%)
Occasional:	569	(59.6%)
1-2/day:	210	(22.0%)
More than 2/day:	49	(5.1%)

24. Do you exercise? 946 replies

No:	407	(43.3%)
Yes:	538	(56.9%)

25. What form of contraception do you use? 251 replies

Oral contraceptives:	2	(0.8%)
Foam:	7	(2.8%)
"Sponge":	3	(1.2%)
Diaphragm:	12	(4.8%)
Condom:	27	(10.8%)
Tubal ligation:	83	(33.1%)
Vasectomy:	27	(10.8%)

26. What is your major source of information on menopause? 452 replies

Books:	101	(22.3%)
Magazines:	149	(33.0%)
Pamphlets:	20	(4.4%)
Doctor:	94	(20.8%)
Friends:	60	(13.3%)
Mother:	23	(5.1%)
TV/Radio:	5	(1.1%)

27. What issue regarding menopause most interests you? 873 replies

Estrogen replacement:	197	(26.2%)
Breast cancer:	95	(12.6%)
Ovarian cancer:	15	(1.6%)
Osteoporosis:	310	(41.2%)
Uterine cancer:	18	(2.4%)
Pregnancy:	12	(1.6%)

28. Does the man in your life understand menopause? 873 replies

No:	131	(15.0%)
Yes:	428	(49.0%)
Not applicable:	314	(36.0%)

29. Have you worked outside the home? 861 replies

No:	80	(9.3%)
Yes:	761	(90.7%)

30. Are you working now? 956 replies

No:	184	(19.2%)
Yes:	772	(80.8%)
Part-time:	218	(28.6%)
Full-time:	544	(71.3%)

31. Educational level: (960 replies)

High school:	24	(2.5%)
Some college:	126	(13.1%)
College grad:	345	(35.9%)
Graduate work:	157	(16.4%)
(some, no degree)		
Master's:	221	(23.6%)
Doctorate:	83	(8.6%)

32. Annual family income: (747 replies)

0–$10,000	3	(0.4%)
$10,000–$25,000	44	(5.9%)
$25,000–$50,000	229	(30.7%)
$50,000–$100,000	295	(39.5%)
More than $100,000	176	(23.6%)

33. Personal annual income: (828 replies)

0–$10,000	210	(25.4%)
$10,000–$25,000	213	(25.7%)
$25,000–$50,000	274	(33.1%)
$50,000–$100,000	97	(11.7%)
More than $100,000	33	(4.0%)

Demographically, our group of respondents is well-educated and well off. Almost 85 percent are college educated. The majority (73 percent) are married. Eighty percent are currently employed. Nearly 94 percent have family incomes over $25,000 annually; 62 percent have family incomes over $50,000. However, 25 percent of our respondents have personal incomes of less than $25,000, implying that even this highly educated, preponderantly working group of women is highly dependent upon the spouse's income.

The majority of women reported a variety of menopausal symptoms. Sixty-three percent reported either mild or severe hot flashes; 38 percent reported vaginal dryness. Forty-nine percent had experienced some stress incontinence, although only 4.7 percent considered it severe. Fifty-eight percent reported problems with weight gain over the perimenopausal years, and 47 percent found depression to be a problem, although only 6.5 percent reported it as severe. What was interesting about the comments is that the women who reported few symptoms seemed to think these body changes mainly psychological, whereas the women who had experienced physical difficulties were firmly convinced they were purely physical.

The women gynecologists did not differ significantly in terms of reported symptoms, so knowledge itself does not offer any magic protection!

However, women gynecologists *did* report a number of differences. More of them had had hysterectomies (44.4 percent vs. 29.7 percent). More gynecologists had had their ovaries removed (25.5 percent vs. 13.4 percent). Surprisingly, fewer gynecologists had had mammograms (57.7% vs. 62.4%), not a particularly wide margin but nonetheless we had expected a much higher proportion of these knowledgeable women with good access to medical care to avail themselves of screening mammography. More gynecologists took hormones in general (62 percent vs. 26.7 percent), and in particular estrogen pills (26.9% vs. 12.2%) or estrogen/progesterone pills (26.9 percent vs. 9.4%).

Overall, the group's health habits were good. Only 5.1 percent reported consuming more than two drinks per day. Eighty-one percent are nonsmokers; 57 percent exercise regularly. However, 57 percent reported they were overweight, although only 15 percent were severely (more than 30 pounds) obese. Most of the women reported their major source of health information to be magazines (33 percent) and books (22 percent); doctors (21 percent) and friends (13 percent) followed closely behind, with mothers (5 percent) and TV/Radio (1.1 percent) being less common sources of information. Again, in many ways the most revealing parts of the survey were the comments written in the margin and in separate notes, often expressing frustration with a society little attuned to the needs of midlife women—and hope that we could bring to light some of the real physical problems associated with midlife while laying to rest some of the myths.

INDEX